Engineering catastrophes

Related titles from Woodhead's materials list:

Fatigue in railway structures
ISBN-13: 978-185573-740-2
ISBN-10: 1-85573-740-X

Fatigue strength of welded structures
ISBN-13: 978-185573-506-4
ISBN-10: 1-85573-506-7

Cumulative damage of welded joints
ISBN-13: 978-185573-938-3
ISBN-10: 1-85573-938-0

Emerging infrastructure materials
ISBN-13: 978-185573-943-7
ISBN-10: 1-85573-943-7

Analysis and design of plated structures Volume I: Stability
ISBN-13: 978-185573-967-3
ISBN-10: 1-85573-967-4

Details of these books and a complete list of Woodhead's materials titles can be obtained by:

- Visiting our web site at www.woodheadpublishing.com
- Contacting Customer Services (e-mail: sales@woodhead-publishing.com; fax: +44 (0) 1223 893694; tel: +44 (0) 1223 891358 ext 30; address: Woodhead Publishing Limited, Abington Hall, Abington, Cambridge CB1 6AH, England)

Engineering catastrophes

Causes and effects of major accidents

Third edition

JOHN LANCASTER

CRC Press
Boca Raton Boston New York Washington, DC

WOODHEAD PUBLISHING LIMITED
Cambridge England

Published by Woodhead Publishing Limited, Abington Hall, Abington
Cambridge CB1 6AH, England
www.woodheadpublishing.com

Published in North America by CRC Press LLC, 6000 Broken Sound
Parkway, NW, Suite 300, Boca Raton, FL 33487, USA

First edition 1996, Abington Publishing
Reprinted in paperback 1997
Second edition 2000, Abington Publishing and CRC Press LLC
Third edition 2005, Woodhead Publishing Ltd and CRC Press LLC
© 2005, Woodhead Publishing Ltd
The author has asserted his moral rights.

British Library Cataloguing in Publication Data
A catalogue record for this book is available from the British Library.

Library of Congress Cataloging in Publication Data
A catalog record for this book is available from the Library of Congress.

Woodhead Publishing ISBN-13: 978-1-84569-016-8 (book)
Woodhead Publishing ISBN-10: 1-84569-016-8 (book)
Woodhead Publishing ISBN-13: 978-1-84569-081-6 (e-book)
Woodhead Publishing ISBN-10: 1-84569-081-8 (e-book)
CRC Press ISBN-10: 0-8493-9878-9
CRC Press order number: WP9878

The publishers' policy is to use permanent paper from mills that operate a
sustainable forestry policy, and which has been manufactured from pulp which is
processed using acid-free and elementary chlorine-free practices.
Furthermore, the publishers ensure that the text paper and cover board used
have met acceptable environmental accreditation standards.

Typeset by SNP Best-set Typesetter Ltd., Hong Kong
Printed by TJ International Ltd, Padstow, Cornwall, England

Contents

Preface to third edition

There is a widely held, but rarely stated theory of accidents, according to which each and every mishap has a cause, and that safety may best be assured by discovering these causes and preventing their occurrence. The first edition of this book was written from such a viewpoint, with particular emphasis on mechanical failure. One reviewer of this edition pointed out, quite correctly, that the human factor had been ignored. Accordingly an extra chapter was added to the second edition, where the manner in which human behaviour affected the incidence of accidents was examined. As a result of this and much subsequent work, it has become evident that human behaviour is not just a factor that affects improved safety and economic growth, but that it entirely controls such developments. In this third edition, therefore, the final chapter of the second edition has been omitted, and Chapters 1 and 2 have been entirely rewritten so as to provide a method of analysing the records of accident and all-cause mortality rates and their decrease with the passage of time, to show their relationship with levels of economic development and economic growth rates, and to make suggestions about the ways in which such processes may be linked.

The picture that emerges is a very strange one. It would seem that human beings inhabit, simultaneously, two separate worlds, between which there is no direct communication. Firstly, there is the conscious world: that of politics, entertainment, art, science and technology. The second world, of which we are but dimly aware, comprises the subconsciously-directed activity of large populations, which results in economic growth and the reduction of mortality rates due to physical and biological accidents. Evidence for the existence of the second world lies in the relevant historical records, such as those examined in the first two chapters of this book. These indicate a remarkably well-ordered, self-regulated activity and, in the case of falling accident rates, one which is self-initiated. There is a close link between economic growth and the fall in accident rates, such that both may be regarded as aspects of human development as a whole.

These concepts are difficult to understand and accept because they relate to human activities that are subconsciously guided, whereas it is generally considered that human actions are guided by conscious, rational thought. It may therefore be useful to look at a specific case.

Records for fatality rates due to accidents on British roads date back to 1926. From 1926 to 1934 these death rates showed a steady annual rise. Then in 1934 there was an abrupt change. The death rate from road accidents began to fall exponentially. The conscious world played no part in this event and was not, at the time, aware that it had occurred. Evidently, it was the result of a subconsciously motivated change in the behaviour of the vehicle driver population.

Subsequently (except for a temporary upward surge during the 1939–45 War) road fatality rates have fallen at between 4.5% and 5.5% annually, and in a very well-ordered manner. It is suggested in Chapter 1 that this fall is due to the development of collective skill amongst the population of drivers. Such a process involves interactions between millions of individuals, and would be expected to show the observed regularity.

The motivation for the initiation and continuance of the exponential fall of fatality rates must surely be the instinct for self-preservation. Two factors could influence the pace at which the accident rate falls: the nature of the activity; and the native ability of the population concerned. There are also indications that in some circumstances the perception of risk may have a controlling effect.

During the period after 1934 there were numerous attempts by various British governments and their agencies to improve road safety by legislation and punitive action. The record shows that in one instance (the law that made it compulsory to wear seat belts) there followed an *increase* in pedestrian deaths, but that overall such legislation had no measurable effect on road deaths. This result is consistent with the model of fatality rate reduction presented here, and also with the idea that there is little or no communication between the conscious and subconscious worlds.

The pattern of events described above for road deaths in Britain is similar to that for most industries and modes of transport considered in this book. Industry and transport in other developed countries almost certainly follow a similar course. An exception is the oil industry, where fatality rates in exploration and financial loss due to accidents in oil refineries follow a fluctuating course, as described in Chapter 2.

It is proposed in the text that scientific and technological developments represent a permissive factor. They make improvements in productivity and safety possible, but the pace of such improvements is set by the population concerned. It may well be that this principle applies to the initiation of the fall in accident rates. In earlier times the relatively rapid fall characteristic of the twentieth century did not occur. Where records go sufficiently far back in time, they show a period where the rate is rising, flat or slowly declining. In England and Wales the mortality rate from all causes started to decline rapidly for children and young adults during the early 1860s. This was the initiation of an exponential decline which has continued. The 1850s and 1860s were decades when 'germs' – the living agents of contagious disease – were discovered and their existence generally accepted. Thus, it became possible to combat disease and the population took advantage of this fact, albeit subconsciously. In this instance, scientific knowledge may well have been the trigger for the initiation of the exponential fall.

In the nature of things, it is not possible to speak with certainty about the motivation of subconsciously-guided processes. But it would seem reasonable to suppose that both the initiation and the continuance of the exponential fall in fatality rates must have received their impetus from the human instinct for survival. This is especially the case for mortality from all causes. The record here is most remarkable. For several millennia, since the beginning of civilisation, mankind has been cursed by the prevalence of infectious disease, which has caused innumerable tragedies due to the premature deaths of children, and young men and women. Then, in the relatively short period of 100 years between 1860 and 1960, this menace was eliminated in the developed countries by simple acts of hygiene on the part of the population and by engineering developments. The conquest of infectious disease must rank as one of the greatest of human achievements, but it took place mainly in the subconscious sphere, and has little recognition in the conscious world.

Finally, there remains one question that cannot be answered here. If economic growth and mortality reduction are self-regulating, what, apart from the defence of the realm and the maintenance of internal peace, should be the responsibilities of governments? In other words, what are the essential matters that require regulation, and what would be best left in the hands of the population at large?

Preface to second edition

In the first edition of this book, the incidence of accidents to vehicles and structures was considered primarily in relation to mechanical breakdown, on the one hand, or to human error, on the other. The effect of collective human behaviour was noted in specific cases, but in general this important topic was not covered. In order to redress the balance, a new chapter entitled 'The human factor' has been added. In this chapter loss and fatality rates are reviewed in general terms, together with their relationship to large-scale events such as war and the trade cycle. Historical data on road and rail accidents, which are particularly relevant to this subject, have been added.

In most industries and modes of transport, casualty and loss rates (annual number of deaths in road accidents per 10 000 licensed vehicles, for example) fall with time. Technological improvements have undoubtedly contributed largely to such beneficial changes. However, the effect of human behaviour cannot be ignored and there are instances in which the human factor appears to have had a large and predominant effect.

One such case is that of railways in Britain. Prior to the Second World War, the number of passengers killed annually in train accidents had fallen to a low level. During and immediately after the war, however, these fatality numbers rose almost ten-fold, and remained high until 1953, after which they started to fall. There was no physical change in the railway system that could explain this sharp rise, which must have resulted from a change in behaviour on the part of railway workers. Disaffection amongst manual workers – the 'British disease' – was widespread in the post-war era, and the railways seem to have suffered accordingly.

In the previous edition of this book, much space was expended in an attempt to discover why, in a safety-conscious industry such as hydrocarbon processing, capital losses should be increasing instead of diminishing. Time has now provided an answer. After a long period of increase, capital losses in oil refineries fell from 558.7 million US dollars (US$) in 1992 to US$ 72.4 million in 1993, and have remained low up to the latest recorded figure of US$ 12.1 million in 1996. There is no possibility of any significant change in the relevant hardware between 1992 and 1993, so once again human behaviour (in this instance that of refinery operators) must have been responsible for the change. Even with contemporary levels of automation and computer control it is possible to operate process plant in a more risky or less risky fashion, but the size of the reduction, and the fact that it occurred in plants scattered over the whole world, is quite remarkable. The timing is not so remarkable; this was a period of recession, when loss and fatality rates tend to fall. It had nothing to do with throughput; consumption of crude oil remained steady during the recession.

Apart from such relatively dramatic developments, there is a general correlation between measures of economic growth and those of casualty and loss rates. For example in Britain (and no doubt elsewhere) fatality rates in road accidents fell less rapidly during the economic boom of the 1980s and dipped sharply during the subsequent recession. Accidents in manufacturing industry followed a similar pattern. Such indicators may be taken as a measure of the level of activity amongst the population of the nation in question. Amongst developed countries the relevant figures are broadly similar; the per capita gross domestic product is of the same order of magnitude, and although growth rates are characteristic of particular countries, they fall within a fairly narrow band. Worldwide, however, this is not so, and the per capita gross domestic product of the richest nations is over a thousand times greater than that of the poorest. Here, too, there is a correlation between economic and safety indicators; fatality rates in road accidents are highest in the poorer countries, and vice versa. Again, the ratio between the highest and lowest figures is in the region of one thousand.

The mechanisms that determine the levels of safety and economic growth are a matter for speculation. Clearly, they involve the interaction of large numbers of individuals, either directly or indirectly through technical improvements. Thus, the skill of drivers improves as a result of collective experience, whilst at the same time the vehicles and roads become safer. The effectiveness of these changes will depend on the native ability and temperament of the population concerned.

The final conclusion is that collective human behaviour is the predominant factor in determining fatality and loss rates. The earlier view, that improved safety results from a reduction in the incidence of human error by technical change may provide a useful model in specific cases, but it is not generally applicable. The incidence of human error may change of its own accord; it may decrease through the acquisition of skills, or it may increase through the development of negative attitudes of mind. Technical change is itself the product of human inventiveness and effort. So the whole process is governed by human behaviour and its direction and rate are determined internally by mechanisms which are, at present, little understood. Positive economic growth is linked to falling accident rates and their respective levels result from the history of the population concerned. The trend is positive, although marred from time to time by a South Sea Bubble or a 'Titanic' catastrophe.

One thing is certain: in a peaceful democratic country it is not possible for an individual, be that individual king, queen, president or prime minister, to intervene directly so as to change the rate or direction of such processes. There is no chain of command that would enable orders to be conveyed to the populace at large. Nor is it likely, supposing such orders were received, that they would be obeyed. It is characteristic of loss and casualty rates where there is a large population that they display a lot of inertia, such that over a long period of time the reduction in the casualty or loss rate will either remain constant or will vary in a regular manner. This behaviour is to be expected from a network that has millions of connections, and by the same token it is not likely to be affected by exhortation or orders from individuals. Governments may contribute to safety by practical measures such as better roads or improved harbours, but they cannot improve safety by regulation, or increase the economic growth rate by passing a law to that effect.

Preface to first edition

One of the privileges of the great, said Jean Giraudoux, is to witness catastrophes from a terrace. Giraudoux, who died in 1944, was a writer and diplomat, but he was not much of a prophet. Television has made nonsense of his words; today, it is the privilege of the multitude to witness catastrophes from an armchair. Come flood, fire, famine, storm, tempest, earthquake, volcanic eruptions or tidal waves, if the cameras can get there we will see it. No longer is it necessary to imagine suffering caused by disaster; it is there before us.

According to data collected by the United Nations, the cost of reconstruction following natural disasters, and the numbers of people killed or seriously affected by them, has risen during the last 30 years by an average of about 6% per year. This is to be compared with an annual population growth rate of 2%. Nobody knows why the effects of these catastrophes are increasing at such a rapid rate, but it is certain that they apply most severely to those countries that can least afford the cost. The years 1994–2004 have been declared 'the decade for natural disaster reduction'.

In the nineteenth century a new type of man-made catastrophe appeared. This was the start of the period of mass transportation, when railway accidents could, and sometimes did, result in large numbers of deaths. At the start of the century ships were relatively small so not many lives were lost when a single vessel foundered. Tonnages increased quite rapidly, however, and this period of growth culminated with the loss of over 1500 lives when the *Titanic* sank.

During the same period factories powered by steam engines grew in number and in size, as did the number of industrial accidents. One of the scandals of this period was the death rate due to boiler explosions. These peaked in about 1900 and then mercifully declined.

In the twentieth century we have seen the development of air transport, and the increasing size of aircraft has meant that a single loss could result in hundreds of deaths. Another big development has been in ferry transport, particularly roll-on, roll-off vehicle ferries. Here there have been some widely publicised catastrophes, notably the *Herald of Free Enterprise* and the *Estonia*. The worst ever shipping disaster was the sinking of a passenger ferry in the Philippines, with the loss of over 4000 lives.

More recently the search for oil and gas on the continental shelf has led to a completely new type of maritime activity. On mobile platforms in the North Sea it is a particularly dangerous one, comparable with deep-sea fishing so far as risk is concerned.

So where do we stand? Does the onward march of technology mean that more people are facing greater hazards, or is it otherwise?

It is the purpose of this book to try to answer the question by looking at the historical record of casualty and loss. War and pestilence have been excluded and natural catastrophes are dealt with only in general terms, except, for reasons that will be set forth later, in the case of earthquakes. Most emphasis is on accidents to man-made objects and where possible the records that are kept on a worldwide basis will be used. It must be recognised, however, that such records refer almost entirely to ships, aircraft and so forth that are made in and operated by industrial countries.

I have tried as far as possible to avoid technical jargon. In particular the use of acronyms, except for a few old friends, has been avoided. This tiresome and unnecessary practice afflicts offshore technology more than most, such that some parts of Lord Cullen's report on the *Piper Alpha* disaster are incomprehensible, at least to the ordinary reader. Every effort has been made here to call a spade a spade.

Many of the disasters recorded in this book took place before the current (SI) system of units came into use. Where this is the case, the units quoted in the text are those given in the contemporary documents. A conversion table is provided in Appendix 2 in order that these older units may be transposed, should this be so required.

Acknowledgements

The author wishes to express his thanks for information provided by staff of The Health and Safety Executive and that of The Office for National Statistics. Paul Wilkinson of the Railway Inspectorate provided much information on passenger safety. His publisher gave unfailing support, and Rob Burleigh extracted large quantities of data from a CD kindly supplied by the Mortality Section of The Office for National Statistics. Ian Sheriff, of Det Norske Veritas, provided valuable information about offshore losses. As always, the author is much indebted to his wife for translating an ungainly scrawl into presentable material.

CHAPTER I

Analysing casualty records

How big is a catastrophe?

It is natural to associate the word 'catastrophe' with some large-scale event such as the collison of two passenger aircraft, or the destruction by fire of a major off-shore oil platform like *Piper Alpha*. In the case of fatal accidents, however, it is not so simple. Where does one draw the line? Must there be one hundred deaths, or 50 or 20? There is no good answer to this question. Indeed, the premature accidental death of a single person is a tragedy for family and friends, and may have dire financial consequences. Therefore much of this book will be concerned with fatal accidents regardless of their scale.

A great deal of data concerning accidents has accumulated during the nineteenth and twentieth centuries. Early contributors to this collection in Britain were the Census Office (now the Office for National Statistics), which first produced figures for mortality in 1841, Her Majesty's Inspector of Factories, and the Railway Inspectorate. The introduction of the motor vehicle at the beginning of the twentieth century resulted in a sharp rise in casualities on roads. In Europe and North America government departments provided records of these. In Britain, the Office for National Statistics gives figures for accident mortality, including those that are due to road traffic, from 1901. Lloyd's Register of Shipping publishes an annual statistical summary for losses from the world's commercial fleet,[1] the first copy of which was issued in 1891. The Boeing Company has performed a similar service for jet passenger aircraft since 1964.[2] Although accidents are responsible for only a small proportion of deaths, they are a matter of universal concern, and if public interest fades from time to time, it is soon reawakened by some newsworthy disaster.

In making an analytical study of such material, the first step is to establish units. Time is the most straightforward; one year is almost universally taken as the unit. Seasonal variations in the number of accidents are not uncommon and the use of annual data eliminates this variable.

The quantitative measure for accidents must surely be the rate, that is, the annual number of deaths divided by the number of people employed in the activity concerned; in short, annual deaths/population. The mortality rate in a particular country conforms to this model, whether mortality is considered as that due to all causes or as that due to accidents. Records may not provide a direct measure of the mortality rate; for example, in the case of shipping, Lloyd's casualty reports give the percentage loss of ships from the world fleet. However, this figure could reasonably be taken as a measure of the proportional loss of ships' crews. Numbers of people killed in train accidents may be related to the number of journeys, this latter figure being a measure of the population of rail passengers.

Whatever the merits or demerits of such measures, it is a fact that during the twentieth century mortality and loss rates fell in the majority of cases and, moreover, the pattern of their decline was similar. It is therefore possible to analyse the historical records of accident rates in general, regardless of the activity to which they relate.

In analysing the accident record it is necessary to make use of various mathematical techniques. Details are given in Appendix 1. Only the results will be given in the main text.

Perspectives

Before proceeding with an examination of the historical data, it will be instructive to look at some figures for accidents as a whole. For the year 2000 in England and Wales the total number of accidental deaths (excluding suicide and homicide) was 11 149, this being 2.08% of the number of deaths from all causes. The document from which these figures are taken[3] allocates deaths in one of four categories, three of which are causes, whilst one (transport) is an activity. The allocation is shown as a bar chart in Fig. 1.1, from which it will be seen that falling (from a ladder, for example) is the commonest cause of accidental death. This category covers all activities other than transport, including industry, sport and domestic life, as does the category 'fire'. Fatalities from both these causes decreased throughout the twentieth century.

Transport accounted for nearly one-third of accidental deaths at the beginning of the twenty-first century. Of these, 92% are the result of road traffic accidents. Rail and other forms of transport cause relatively few casualties. Since 1900 the increase in range and speed of both air and road transport has been dramatic, and in both cases it has been necessary not only to learn how to operate the individual vehicle, but also to develop systems whereby the risk of collision is minimised. The success of this learning process is evidenced by the reduction in loss and fatality rates as discussed below.

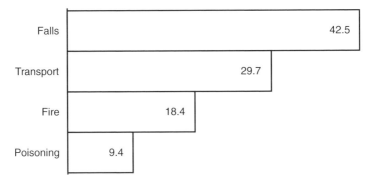

1.1 Causes of accidental death in England and Wales for the year 2000.[3] Inset figures are percentages of the total.

The trend curve for casualty rates: the normal case

Figure 1.2 plots the annual percentage loss in numbers of ships from the world fleet for the period 1891 to 1999. For clarity, data points are shown at ten-year intervals. The solid line in Fig. 1.2 is the trend curve for the set of shipping loss data points. It may be determined using the following procedure:

1   Take the natural logarithms (logarithms to base e) of the loss rates.
2   Plot the resulting figures against the corresponding year dates.
3   Determine the equation of the line that gives the best fit to these data pairs. This equation will take the form

$$\ln r = bt + \text{constant} \qquad [1.1]$$

4   Take the antilogarithm of this equation to obtain the equation of the trend curve

$$r = ae^{bt} \qquad [1.2]$$

where a is another constant, t represents time and b is the slope of the $\ln r$ versus time line. In the case of the shipping losses portrayed in Fig. 1.2, a = 7.99 and b = −0.026, time being measured in anno domini (1891, 1910 etc.). Details of the procedure are given in Appendix 1 but a scientific calculator can be used to obtain a and b directly from the raw data.

The form of this curve is exponential. It is a basic characteristic of an exponential curve that the proportional gradient is constant. In the present case

$$1/r \, dr/dt = b \qquad [1.3]$$

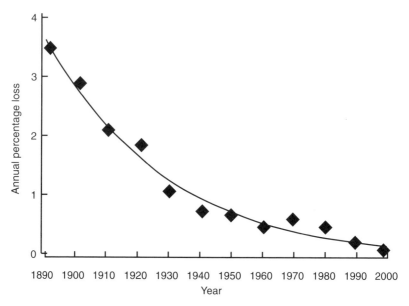

1.2 The percentage of the total number of ships in the world's commercial fleet that was lost annually between the years 1890 and 2000.[1]

Thus, b is the proportional gradient of the loss rate trend curve. The dimension of b is 1/(time) and since in this book the unit of time is 1 year, this dimension is 1/(year). The value of b is therefore independent of the units (annual percentage loss, annual fatality rate per million population, etc.). 'Proportional gradient' is an awkward designation and its meaning is not immediately obvious. In later sections of this book the term 'decrement' is used as an alternative. Decrement is the opposite of increment and means the fact or process of decreasing. Here it will be quantified to mean the annual proportional or percentage reduction in the casualty rate. Thus for shipping losses the proportional gradient of −0.026 may be represented as an annual decrement of 2.6%. This is an approximation in two respects. First, it implies an annual stepwise change, whereas for the trend curve, and the reality which it represents, the change is continuous. Secondly there is a slight numerical inaccuracy; a proportional gradient of −0.026 causes an annual decrement of 2.566491%. The decrement represents therefore a stepwise model that is accurate enough for yearly time intervals and which is easier to understand than the continuous model. A regression analysis using the exponential model is, however, the best way to organise accident and economic growth rate data and obtain values for the decrement, as is shown in Appendix 1.

Collective skills

It is easy to envisage a growth process because this is a matter of common everyday experience. Trees grow, cities spread, traffic increases and national income rises. There is no such obvious model for the progressive diminution of accident rates that was observed here. However, a possible way out of this difficulty is to suppose that as time goes on, the people concerned become progressively more adept in the avoidance of accidents. In other words, the fall in accident rates is a reflection of an increase in skill on the part of the operators in the industry or mode of transport concerned. It seems reasonable in this connection to speak of collective skill since large numbers of individuals are involved and in many instances they must operate a system, for example drivers of vehicles must observe a set of traffic rules. Thus, we may consider that for any particular activity the collective skill increases exponentially with time. The higher the level of collective skill, the lower the loss rate. And it would be expected that the average annual proportional change in skill would be numerically similar to the corresponding figure for loss rate; the faster that skill improves, the faster loss rates decline. Supposing that these speculations are correct, there will be an inverse relationship between skill and loss rate, both for the absolute value at any given time and for their rate of change with time.

Consider first the effect of time. For the period 1900–83 the national output per head (also known as the per capita gross domestic product) in Britain increased exponentially such that, at constant prices, the proportional gradient b was +0.0126. During the same period, non-transport accident mortality in England and Wales (a good representative sample for Britain as a whole) decreased exponentially with a proportional gradient of −0.010. These figures are numerically similar and both fall at the low end of the range for numerical values of b: this range is typically 0.1–0.6.

In Appendix 1 it is shown that the trend curve equation may be expressed in a non-dimensional from

$$r/\bar{\bar{r}} = e^{b(t-\bar{t})} \tag{1.4}$$

where $\bar{\bar{r}}$ is the geometric mean of the accident rate data and $\bar{t}$ is the arithmetic mean of the time date. In this form it is possible, in principle, to plot all trend curves on the same diagram. In Fig. 1.3 data and trend curves for economic growth and non-transport accident mortality in Britain have been plotted for the period 1950–85. The two curves are almost a mirror image of each other.

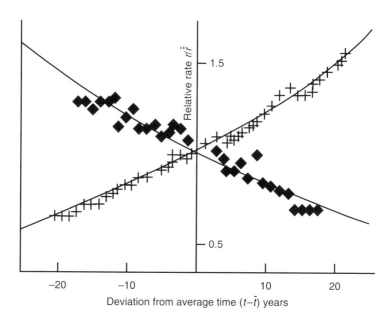

1.3 Data points and non-dimensional trend curves for: ◆, non-transport accident mortality, England and Wales, 1955–85; +, national output per head, Britain, 1955–95.

Accident mortality (excluding transport accidents) was chosen for this comparison because, like economic growth, it reflects the activity of the whole population.

The other inverse relationship proposed earlier is that between skill and fatality rates for different countries at a given point in time. Once again, the national output per head will be taken as the measure of skill. Accident mortality rates are not available for some of the less well-developed nations, so a correlation has been made with road accident fatality rates. Data for road accidents are from the Red Cross[4] and for gross domestic product from the United Nations,[5] both for the period of the early 1990s. A best-fit analysis indicates that the fatality rate is proportional to 1/(national output per head)$^{0.7}$ in line with expectations (Fig. 1.4).

There is a similar hyperbolic relationship between national output per head and the proportion of the relevant population killed or affected by natural disasters (see Chapter 6). More remarkable is that over half a century ago Smeed[6] found that fatality rates in road accidents were related to numbers of vehicles per head of population by an equation almost identical to the one determined here for national output per head. Both these quantities are measures of national prosperity, so it would appear that

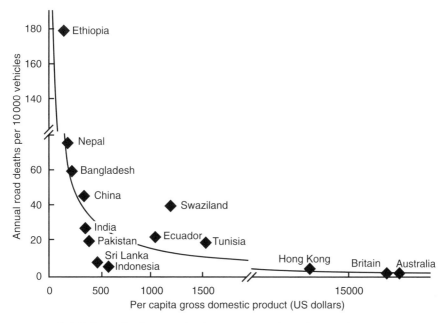

1.4 Relationship between fatality rate in road accidents and per capita gross domestic product for various countries. The scale is altered at the points indicated in order to accommodate extreme data.

the world's economic league table has not changed significantly over the last 50 years.

There is good evidence, therefore, that where an independent measure of skill is available, there is an inverse, quantitative relation between this quantity and loss rates. Moreover, a fall in the loss, fatality or mortality rates is an indication of an increase in the relevant collective skill.

Exponential fall in accident rates

At this stage it will be profitable to look more closely at the normal type of accident record; that is, when there is a steady fall in the casualty rate r, and where a plot of r against time takes the form illustrated in Fig. 1.2.

There are three measurable features relating to such a plot. The first is the trend curve itself and the corresponding relative gradient b. Secondly, data points are scattered relative to the trend curve and the width of the scatter band may be a significant characteristic. The third feature is the frequency distribution of the scatter. The first two of these items are discussed below; frequency distribution is covered in Appendix 1.

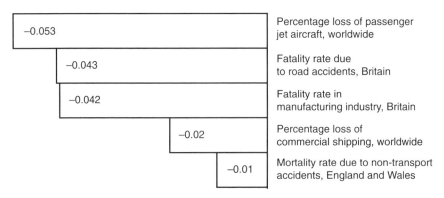

1.5 Proportional gradient of trend curve *b* for various sets of accident data.

The gradient *b*

Figure 1.5 is a bar chart showing typical values of the proportional gradient of the trend curve for various sets of accident data. In all cases the probability of a true correlation is 95% or better. In other words, the curves fit the data very well. Figure 1.5 is for the period 1950–99, except for passenger aircraft losses, which are for 1964–92. There are short-term fluctuations, but for long periods the proportional gradient is usually steady.

The range of values included in Fig. 1.5 is typical of most human activities where the relevant records are available. The higher numerical figures appear to be characteristic of transport and industry, whilst accident mortality for the population as a whole comes at the bottom of the list. Factors that may favour a higher numerical value of the proportional gradient may include small population, ease of communication, specialisation, such that the range of skills to be improved is relatively narrow and higher rates of technological progress. However this may be, the rate of betterment will, in the end, be determined by the willingness and abilities of the population in question.

Variability of casualty rates

In the case of ordinary everyday objects, it is normal practice to consider variation relative to the average or mean value of a particular batch. Consider for example, the day's output of eggs from a poultry farm. This batch will consists of eggs weighing $w_1, w_2, w_3 \ldots w_i, \ldots w_N$ grams, whilst their mean weight is $\bar{w}$ grams. The variance, which is the square of the standard deviation, is then

$$[VAR] - \sigma^2 = 1/N \sum_1^N (w_i - \overline{w})^2 \qquad [1.5]$$

It is also possible to define a non-dimensional or relative form of variance

$$[VAR]_r = \sigma_r^2 = 1/N \sum_1^N (w_i - \overline{w})^2 / \overline{w}^2 \qquad [1.6]$$

Accident rate data differ from this example in two respects: first, the variation is with respect to the trend curve and second, the width of the scatter band diminishes with time. Figure 1.6 illustrates the second feature by comparing the scatter band for British road accident fatality rates during the period 1950–60 with that for 1990–2000. Empirically it is found that the scatter bandwidth is directly proportional to the accident rate predicted by the trend curve r_t. Hence, for any given interval of time it is possible to produce a self-consistent set of scatter data by dividing each deviation by the relevant value of r_t, and in place of $(w_i - \overline{w})$ we have $(r_i - r_{ti})$, where r_i is the actual casualty rate for year i, and r_{ti} is the rate predicted by the trend curve for the same year. The non-dimensional proportional form of this expression is $(r_i - r_{ti})/r_{ti} = (r_i/r_{ti} - 1)$. This procedure produces a set of data $(r_i/r_{ti} - 1)$ from which it is possible to calculate the relative variance and relative standard deviation. It will be convenient to put $r_i/r_{ti} = x_i$ so that

$$[VAR]_r = \sigma_r^2 = 1/N \sum_1^N (x_i - 1)^2 \qquad [1.7]$$

In Fig. 1.6 the scatter boundary lines lie $\pm 2\sigma_r r_t$ on either side of the trend curve. In an ideal case about 95% of data points should fall between these limits. This would seem to be the case here.

The relative standard deviation is a measure of the degree to which data spread relative to the trend curve; it is non-dimensional and may be used to compare different industries and modes of transport. Figure 1.7 shows some relevant values. The factors noted earlier as affecting the proportional gradient b appear to be operative for the relative standard deviation but in the opposite sense; more specialised activities with a smaller population have a wider scatter of data and vice versa. Suppose that the trend curve figure for fatality or loss rate is the target, then it would appear that small populations having the capability of rapid development are likely to miss the target by a wider margin than larger populations where development is at a slower rate.

The mechanical case

Pursuing this mechanistic view of human progress, we may consider the normal case of a population with a falling casualty rate as an interactive

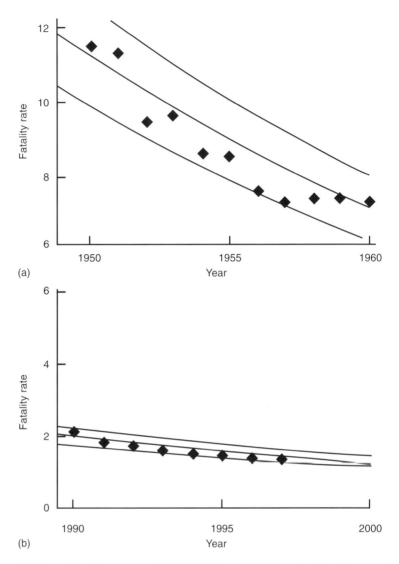

1.6 Annual fatality rate per 10 000 vehicles on British roads: all road users, all vehicles. Shows trend curve for 1950–99 period, together with data points and scatter boundaries formed from (a) 1950–60 and (b) 1990–2000.

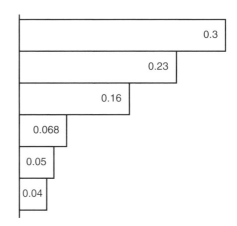

Commercial jet aircraft percentage loss, 1964–92   0.3

Commercial shipping percentage loss, 1950–99   0.23

British manufacturing industry fatality rate, 1950–99   0.16

British roads fatality rate, 1950–99   0.068

Non-transport accident mortality, Britain 1955–99   0.05

National output per head, Britain 1955–99   0.04

1.7 Relative standard deviation for scatter relative to the trend curve: loss and fatality rates and British economic growth, second half of the twentieth century.

system, which is given direction by a positive human attitude towards improvement. Accepting this view, it is of interest to look at the statistical properties of a system that lacks such a driving force, one that is purely mechanical. Gas molecules provide an example of such a system.

Consider a volume of gas at atmospheric temperature and pressure and at rest relating to its surroundings. The gas molecules are very numerous and are in a constant state of motion, and there are frequent collisions between molecules. Such collisions are not mutually destructive; as two molecules approach each other on a collision course, repulsive forces come into play, and each changes its direction of travel and its velocity. Thus, there is an interchange of energy and as a result of such interactions there is a steady distribution of velocities. Now the components of such velocities in a particular direction are statistically similar to the cases examined here; there is a mean value at which data are most numerous, whilst numbers fall off rapidly on either side. For the molecules the average velocity component is zero, since the gas is at rest. There is no change with time, so the quantity b is zero. There is, however, a distribution of velocity components. Appendix 1 shows that the value of the proportional standard deviation is $1/\sqrt{2}$, equal to about 0.707. This figure is substantially higher than those for interactive systems where there is a positive human component. It might therefore be expected that where the human component is negative in character and where there is no improvement in time (the relative gradient of the trend curve b being zero or positive) the relative standard deviation should be close to or exceed 0.707. In Appendix 1 it is shown that this may well be the case.

It would seem that the case of molecular velocity components represents a neutral condition, whose statistical properties lie between those of two types of human interactive systems, one where safety improves with time and another where it does not. This result is consistent with the mechanistic view of safety improvement which was adopted earlier in this section.

The learning process

Earlier in this chapter it was proposed that the observed fall in casualty rates was the result of the development of collective skills on the part of the population in question; the more adeptly an action is performed, the less frequently are accidents likely to occur. It is pertinent, therefore, to examine the circumstances surrounding such developments. As a first step, consider the nature of populations for which accident data are available and, in particular, those considered in this chapter.

These populations fall into one of three categories: international, national and sub-national. The international category comprises aircraft and shipping. In both these categories a common set of rules for avoiding collision has developed. Likewise there is a common technology and there is a tendency for increasing standardisation (in procedures and in types of vehicle, for example) as time goes on. There is another international group – hydrocarbon processing. This activity, which is considered in Chapter 2, also has a common technology. In all three cases the human population (of aircrew, ships' crew and process plant operators) is relatively small and the nationalities are diverse, but the common features justify their treatment as statistical entities.

For national populations, the three records most relevant to this book are those for economic growth, accident mortality and mortality that is due to all causes. The relevant populations are relatively large and activities very diverse. Within each national population there are activities for which accident statistics are available, notably road transport, air transport and the various branches of industry.

For the learning process itself it is profitable to compare the aircraft population with that of road transport drivers. Airline pilots undergo a lengthy and rigorous period of training, at the end of which they are subject to a qualification test. In the course of normal operations retraining is required for significant changes such as new aircraft or new routes. They are also given periodic medical examinations. By contrast the driver of a private car is not, in Britain, required to pass other than a quite rudimentary driving test and is not normally subject to any further testing or training. During operations, airline pilots are in verbal communication with ground staff and, where necessary, with each other. Their land-based counterpart, by contrast, has only the crudest forms of mutual contact: the flashing of lights, sounding of horns, gestures and so forth. Nevertheless, road accident fatality rates in Britain decline almost as fast as do aircraft losses and, in the case of aircraft, the scatter band of the loss rate is broader.

It is not intended to suggest that training and qualification of airline pilots is unnecessary; on the contrary, their responsibilities are such as to justify all such activity. It is, however, clear that the development of collective skills occurs without any formal training and, indeed, without verbal communication between the individuals concerned. Moreover, the improvement in safety takes place without these same individuals being aware of the fact. In the case of fatality rates on British roads, the proportional gradient b is -0.043. This means that on average, fatality rates fall by about 4% annually. But no motorist ever says to him- or herself, 'this coming year I am going to kill 4% fewer of my fellow road users than I did last year'. The process of skill development is one which requires neither verbal communication nor conscious effort. It is in fact the normal result of the interactions in a human population that is pursuing either a specific activity, such as driving vehicles, or a more generalised one, such as earning daily broad.

If, it may be asked, skill development proceeds at its own pace, what role does technological progress play in the reduction of casualty rates? It has been shown (Fig. 1.4) that for the same level of vehicle technology, road traffic fatality rates can vary by nearly $200:1$. On the other hand, it would hardly be possible to maintain contemporary levels of safety and comfort if we were equipped only with stone tools. The answer would appear to be that technological development is an enabling factor. Such changes make economic progress and safety improvement possible, but the speed thereof is determined by the human factors that were set out earlier. It is possible to fly to the moon and back, but commercial trips are some way ahead.

A useful comparison with the role of technology is that of the gardener who wishes to train a plant to climb up a wall. To do so he or she fastens panels of wooden trellis ahead of the plant. Sometimes these will be large pieces (the invention of railways, or of the internal combustion engine, for example), sometimes small, but always ahead. In the meantime the plant ascends at a steady pace, purposefully but unconsciously. This is not too bad a representation; for example, in the case of road traffic, the gardener stands for the automobile engineers, crashworthiness experts, highway constructors and maintenance staff and so on and the plant growth is the development of skill on the part of the driver population. However, walls are limited in height, but, to date, there appears to be no such limitation on technological or human development.

Perturbations

In the preceding discussion it has been implicitly assumed that the statistical measures derived from economic growth and casualty rate data are more or less constant over substantial periods of time. This is indeed the case for the second half of the twentieth century, but during the first half there was much political instability, resulting in two world wars, and these events are reflected in the casualty records. Figure 1.8 shows data for Britain during the period immediately before, during and immediately after the Second World War. The data are for output per head, fatality rates in factories and fatality rates on roads. The period covered is 1934–50. The trend curve shown has been calculated after excluding figures for the years 1939–44, inclusive. These three diagrams are remarkably similar, reinforcing the view that accident rates and economic progress result from the same process. In this instance a burst of economic activity is accompanied by an increase in the casualty rate. Other, but less extreme examples of such a linkage will be noted in Chapter 2.

The other notable features of these diagrams is that when the war was over, the relevant rate did not return to the pre-war level, but fell to a level which it would have reached had there been no war and the trend curve

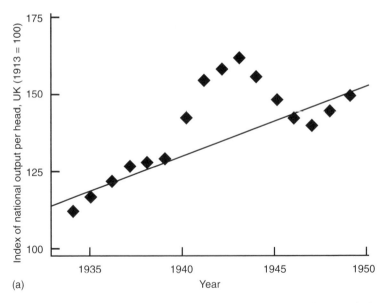

(a)

1.8 Economic output and casualty rates in Britain before, during and after the 1939–45 war. (a) Index of output per head at constant prices, based on 1913 index = 100. (b) Fatality rate per million employees in manufacturing industry. (c) Fatality rate per 10 000 licensed vehicles, all road users.

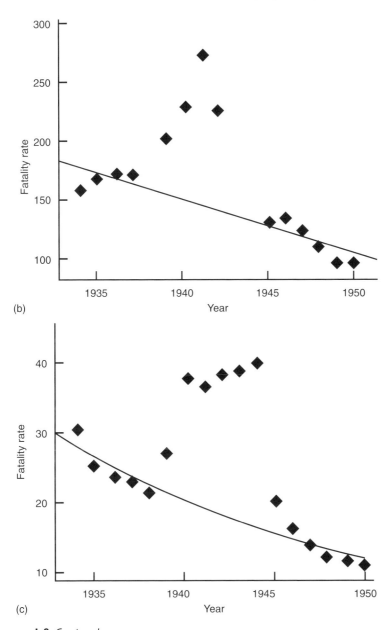

(b)

(c)

1.8 *Continued*

had continued uninterrupted. It is as though during the war all the clocks ran wild, but somewhere there was a hidden timepiece that told the correct time, to which the wild clocks eventually conformed. Passenger fatality rates on British railways, discussed in Chapter 2, follow a similar course. After rising to a high level in the post-war years, these rates fell exponentially to a level predicted by the pre-war trend curve. These are uncomfortable facts that do not fit well into a rational framework.

A second type of perturbation that appears to have no connection with political instabilities is the cyclic tendency. Proportional deviations from the trend curve fall alternately on the positive and negative side, sometimes in quite a regular fashion. Figure 1.9 shows three such cases. The curves shown on this diagram are sinusoidal and have been fitted by eye. The alternation of boom and slump in national output is, of course, notorious. As a rule these ups and downs are usually in phase, at least amongst English-speaking countries. Figure 1.9 shows that shipping losses were also in phase with the trade cycle. This observation is in line with the wartime data: casualty rates increase during economic boom times. The reckless free-spender alternates with the cautious miser.

Cause and effect

A widespread and practical view about accidents is that each and every one has a cause, and that by identifying and eliminating such causes, the incidence of accidents may be reduced. Accidents to aircraft, in particular, are the subject of expert investigations, the results of which may prevent a repetition. In the Boeing survey referred to earlier, causes are put into two main classes: air crew (i.e. pilot error) and mechanical failure. Prescriptions to minimise pilot error are already in place. Mechanical failure comes within the jurisdiction of engineers. Accidents in hydrocarbon processing plants are dealt with in a similar manner by the industry itself. On the roads, accident black spots may be identified and appropriate changes made.

The first edition of this book was written from such a standpoint. One reviewer pointed out, quite correctly, that the human factor was ignored. It now emerges that the human factor is predominant, and that it is the human population (of pilots, drivers, factory workers, etc.) which determines the way in which accident rates diminish or otherwise. Does this mean that conscious efforts to improve safety are futile? Of course not. Any such positive actions are most desirable, but they fall into the same category as technological developments. They help to provide a scope for accident reduction, but the pace thereof is still determined by the human factor, and is not affected by individual technical improvements.

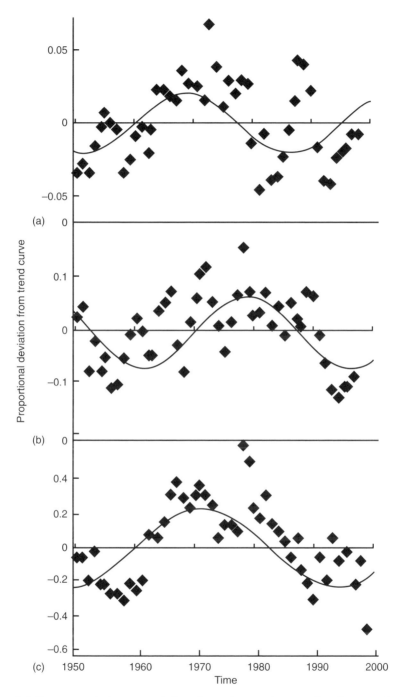

1.9 Proportional deviation of data from the trend curve for the period 1950–2000. (a) National output per head, Britain. (b) Fatality rate per 10 000 vehicles caused by accidents on British roads. (c) Percentage loss of ships from the world's commercial fleet.

Conclusions

1   Examination of available records show that in most instances fatality, loss and accident mortality rates in industry, domestic activities and transport have fallen during the twentieth century. The fall is exponential in character and may be modelled by an equation having the form

$$r = a\mathrm{e}^{bt} \qquad\qquad [1.8]$$

where a and b are constant and t is time counted in years. The quantity b, which is negative for a falling rate, is a measure of the speed with which casualty rates fall and is called the relative gradient.

2   There is a reciprocal relationship between the casualty rate and the economic output, both for their change with time and for values in different countries on a specific date. It is concluded that the changes in both these measures result from the development of collective human skills, such that the population becomes more adept at avoiding accidents.

3   Accident data relating to particular activities (commercial airline operations, for example) are characterised by two quantities: the relative gradient b and the relative standard deviation σ_r, which is a measure of the width of the scatter band of data. Both these quantities are greater for more specialised activities with a smaller population. In such cases, casualty rates fall more quickly and the scatter band of data is wider.

4   These characteristic quantities are determined by the collective actions of the population concerned and are not normally subject to influence from outside. However, in Britain there was a temporary increase both in national output per head and accident rates during both world wars.

References

1. *Lloyd's Casualty Reports*. Annual statistical summary, Lloyd's Register of Shipping, London, published annually.
2. Boeing Commercial Airline Group, *Statistical Summary of Commercial Jet Aircraft Accidents*, Seattle, USA, published annually.
3. *Deaths from Accidents and Violence*, Office for National Statistics, London, published annually.
4. International Federation of Red Cross and Red Crescent Societies, *World Disaster Report*, Oxford University Press, London, 1988.
5. United Nations Yearbook, published annually.
6. Smeed, R.J. 'Some statistical aspects of road safety research', *Roy. J. Statistical Soc. Series A*, 1949 **Part 1** 1–34.

CHAPTER 2

Accident and all-cause mortality: Economic growth

The method established in Chapter 1 will be used here to examine the historical records for accidents in industry and transport, and for mortality due to all causes. Most of the data are for Britain but, where appropriate, international records will be used.

The chapter is divided into three sections. The first deals with those activities where the casualty or loss record conforms to the normal case, that is, when, for most of the period under review, the accident rate falls exponentially with time. The second section is concerned with exceptions, where there are major deviations from a falling rate or where the record does not conform to the normal case at all. In the third section economic growth rates and their relation to the accident record are considered.

Before proceeding, however, it must be recognised that populations are not uniform and that accident rates may vary with age and sex. This factor may be of significance, for example in relation to the 'hidden clock' referred to in Chapter 1.

The effect of sex and age group

Mortality statistics in Britain (and in other industrialised countries) are compiled from death certificates. These documents list age and sex. They also give the cause of death in accordance with the international classification of disease, which includes in its list the various types of accidental physical injury leading to death. It is therefore possible to determine how the risk of accidental death varies across the population. Figure 2.1 illustrates this variation for non-transport fatal accident rates during the year 2000. In calculating mortality rates for this and similar diagrams, the 'population' is that of the age group in question: age groups are 1–4, 5–9, 10–14, 15–19, 20–24, 25–34 and so on up to 75–84. The median of an age group is the age that has an equal numbers of ages above and below it; thus the median of age group 1–4 is 2.5.

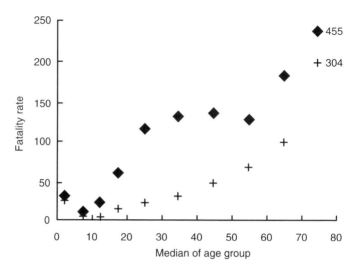

2.1 Accident mortality rate per million population, excluding road deaths, for Britain during the year 2000: the effect of age and sex.[1] ♦, male; +, female.

Transport deaths have been excluded from this compilation on the same grounds as in Chapter 1; namely, that they correlate to numbers of vehicles, not to population numbers.

Clearly, the sexes show different behaviour with respect to accident rates. The female plot indicates a steadily increasing risk of accidental death with increasing age, as would reasonably be expected. Male rates are generally higher, but most particularly so for young men. The difference is more clearly shown in Fig. 2.2, which plots the ratio between male and female fatal accident rates as a function of age. Here there is a sharp peak for the 20–24 age group.

Similar plots for the year 1900 yield qualitatively similar results. Numerically, of course, fatal accident rates were much higher at the beginning of the twentieth century, as was the male/female ratio.

It is tempting to describe the higher fatality rate of young adult males as being due to recklessness. This would be quite wrong. The data plotted in Fig. 2.1 represent averages. A reckless young man is one whose behaviour is more risky than average. The higher accident mortality of young men is normal and has its origins in the genetic makeup of the male.

In Chapter 1 it was observed that during the two world wars of the twentieth century, accident rates tended to rise, sometimes sharply, but when hostilities ceased they reverted, not to the pre-war figure, but to the level at which they would have been had there been no war. It was suggested that there must have been a hidden clock, keeping correct time until peace

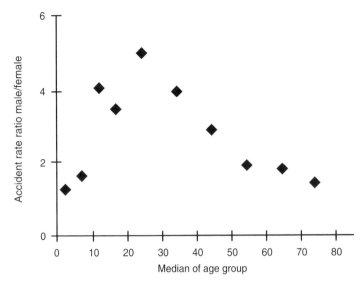

2.2 Fatal accident rate per million population, excluding road deaths for the year 2000: ratio between male and female rates as a function of age.

returned. In fact, the clock is not hidden, but is visible in Fig. 2.1, and comprises females and older males. It is probable that the rise in the civilian mortality rate in wartime was largely due to deaths amongst young men. The bulk of the population proceeds as normal.

Male behaviour may also be responsible for those exceptional cases where casualty rates do not decrease with the passage of time. Where the prevailing attitude is that of enterprising young men, then the change to a falling loss rate may be inhibited. The oil industry (to be discussed later) is a case in point.

There is one other general factor that may affect accident mortality. For either sex, and within any given age group, the level of acceptable risk varies from one individual to another. This human characteristic is not a measurable quantity and does not appear in accident statistics. However, it does have an impact in maritime disasters, as will be described in Chapter 3. Those who are prepared to take greater risks – the bold ones – jump into the sea and are saved, whilst the less bold cling to the wreckage and are drowned. Thus, although in ordinary times brash young men may have a greater likelihood of dying by accident, in emergencies and in human conflicts it may be the other way around.

Industry and transport: the normal case

British manufacturing industry

Published data in the manufacturing area are patchy. From the late nineteenth century onwards figures are given in the annual reports of the factory inspector. This responsibility was taken over by the Health and Safety Executive in 1975. The latter organisation published summaries of this data from 1880 to 1968 and from 1981 to 2000.[2,3] Figures between 1968 and 1981 are missing. Employment statistics were published by the relevant ministry in 1971[3] and more recent figures are held by the Office for National Statistics. However, employment figures for the two world wars are not available, therefore the fatality rate (annual deaths per million employees) is incomplete. There are however enough data to establish trends.[4,5]

Figure 2.3 shows the available data for fatality rate in British factories from 1880 to 2000. For clarity of presentation, five-year averages are plotted.

The figure divides naturally into two parts: before and after the First World War. For the pre-war period the trend line is a best-fit straight line for the data points shown. It indicates an average rise for the fatality rate of about 2% annually.

Earlier, the government of the day had passed numbers of laws and regulations designed to reduce the number of deaths due to accidents in

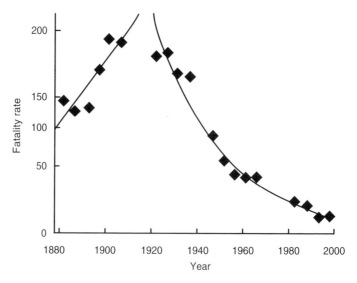

2.3 Annual fatality rate per million employees in British factories, 1880–2000, excluding the two war periods and the years 1969–80.[2–4]

factories. A substantial part of the annual report of the factory inspectorate during this period is concerned with legal actions taken against employers who contravened these Acts. It is evident that such actions failed to arrest the rising trend in the fatality rate that occurred during the late nineteenth and early twentieth century and it is probable that neither the government nor the factory inspectorate were aware of this fact.

The post-war period saw the inception of an exponential fall in fatal accident rates which continued steadily to the beginning of the twenty-first century, with an annual decrement of 3.3%.

During the early part of the First World War, recruitment to the army was voluntary and large numbers of young men joined up. These recruits included factory workers, whose place was taken by women. It will be evident from the previous section that increasing the proportion of females in the factory workforce would reduce the fatality rate. As indicated earlier, fatality rates in British factories during wartime is not known, but numbers of accidental deaths are recorded. These were below 1000 in 1913. During 1914 they fell slightly, increasing by about 100 each year in subsequent war years. Bearing in mind the probability that the number of factory employees must have increased substantially, these increases are modest. It would seem then that the war years constituted a watershed for accidental deaths in British factories. Numbers started to fall in 1921, helped, no doubt, by the post-war economic depression.

This is one instance where the initiation of an exponential fall in casualty rates can be linked to political and economic events. Other such initiations, however, seem to have no such connection.

Air transport

Since 1964 the Boeing Aircraft Company has maintained records of commercial jet aircraft casualties on an international basis. Quantitative data for the early days of passenger flights are entirely lacking. Jet-powered aircraft were first used commercially in the early 1950s when the 'Comet' (whose history is recounted in Chapter 3) came into service. Their use on a wide scale came a decade later, with the introduction of the Boeing 707. The figures compiled by Boeing therefore provide an almost complete record for this type of aircraft.

The Boeing survey provides an analysis of the causes of aircraft accidents. These fall into one of two main categories: air crew, meaning human error, and mechanical failure, which is regarded here as human error at one stage removed. The fate of the early Comet aircraft provides a good example of the second category. Two of these exploded in mid-air owing to a rare catastrophic brittle fracture of the aluminium alloy fuselage. At the time

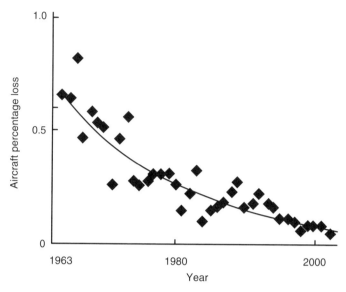

2.4 Percentage of commercial jet aircraft totally lost during the period 1964–2002.[6] Annual decrement 5.7%; relative standard deviation 0.29.

this was ascribed to the designer's use of rectangular window openings, as a result of which excessive stresses built up at the corners. Recently, however, it has emerged that during the construction phase there was difficulty in obtaining a good adhesive joint between the openings and their reinforcing frame and the works manager asked for permission to strengthen the corner areas by riveting. The engineer responsible for construction made this concession. It was from these rivet holes that the fatal cracking originated.

Figure 2.4 shows the percentage loss of jet aircraft for the world's commercial fleet between the years 1964 and 2002. The figures are similar to those for commercial shipping. They start rather higher, but decline more rapidly, the annual decrement being over 5%. The proportional width of the scatter band relative to the trend curve is much the same, about 0.3. Indeed, although ships and aircraft are two very different types of vehicle, their operation has much in common. For example, navigational skill makes a major contribution to safety in both cases.

The risk of being killed in an aircraft accident has likewise fallen quite sharply since 1964, as illustrated in Fig. 2.5. The trend curve value at the beginning of the period was 125 per million departures, more than one in ten thousand. By the end of the century this had been reduced to 23 per million departures. This represents a creditable improvement, but remains

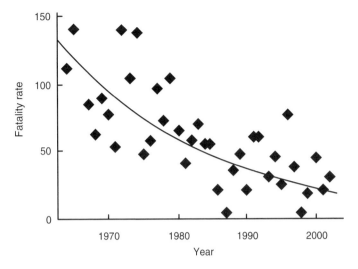

2.5 Annual fatality rate per million departures for passengers and crew of commercial jet aircraft, 1964–2002. The data point for 1966 (fatality rate = 290) has not been plotted but is taken into account in calculating the best-fit curve. Annual decrement 4.7%; relative standard deviation 0.58.

high compared with other forms of bulk passenger transport. During the same period the fatality rate for passengers on British railways was less than one in one hundred million journeys.

British road transport

The mortality rate due to road accidents in Britain varies with age group and sex, in the same way it does for accidents in general; that is to say, the mortality rate for females increases uniformly with age, whereas that for males rises to a peak corresponding to the 20–24 age group, falls and then rises again for the higher age groups. The ratio between male and female road accident mortality rates is almost identical to that for non-transport accidents as shown in Fig. 2.2, with young men in their twenties being about five times more likely to be killed on roads than young women of the same age.

In measuring the variation of fatality risk on roads with time, the rate employed will, as before, be the annual number of deaths divided by the number of registered vehicles. Normally the deaths of all types of road user are included, whilst vehicle numbers are those of all powered two-, three- and four-wheeled vehicles.

Such data are plotted in Fig. 2.6 for the period 1926 (the first date for which figures are available) to 2001. This diagram shows three notable

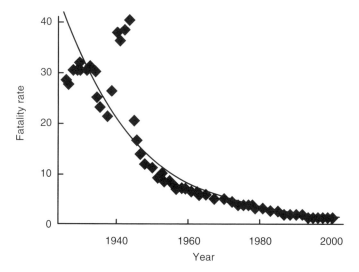

2.6 Annual fatality rate per 10000 vehicles on British roads, 1926–2001, all vehicles, all road users. Annual decrement 4.8%.

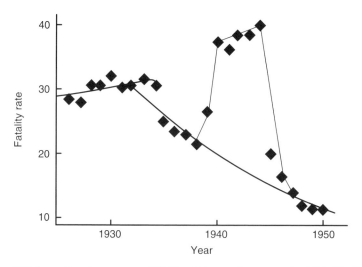

2.7 Annual fatality rate per 10000 vehicles on British roads, 1926–50, all vehicles, all road users. Annual decrement, 1934–50, ignoring war years, 5.4%.

features: an initial period from 1926 to 1934, when there was a rising trend, an exponential fall initiated in 1934 and continuing to 2001, and a series of upward excusions during the Second World War.

Figure 2.7 shows detail for the period 1926–50. In its early days, motoring was a leisure and sporting activity, the record from 1926–34 suggesting that the attitude towards risk was dominated by that of young men. Then, in 1934, there was an abrupt change from an upward trend in the fatality rates to an exponential fall.

The year 1934 was not marked by any major political or other event that might have triggered such a change. However, recovery from the economic collapse of 1929 had started in 1933, when vehicle registrations began to increase, after reaching a low point in 1931 and 1932. There are similarities here to the record for British manufacture, where an increasing fatality rate was arrested at the outbreak of the 1914–18 war and an exponential fall was initiated during the post-war economic recovery. In the present case, a rising trend was interrupted by the 1929 crash and an exponential fall initiated by the recovery after the recession of the 1930s.

It was earlier suggested that the increase in fatal accident rates during wartime is the result of an increase in accidental deaths amongst young men and that amongst the bulk of the population the rate continues to decline in the normal way. It is probable that a similar process occurs in the case of road deaths. The continuity between the pre-war and post-war trend curves lends support to this supposition. It would seem that when hostilities ceased, young men conformed to the reduced fatality rate established by female and older male drivers. Conforming to the majority in this way must be a general human characteristic because there is a regular supply of learner drivers who must eventually conform to contemporary standards.

The seat belt law

The record for casualties on British roads for the period after the Second World War shows a steady exponential fall in the fatality rate, with an annual decrement of nearly 4.5% and a low relative standard deviation of 0.069. The record indicates a steady improvement in safety.

Unaware, or unheeding of this fact, the British parliament passed a law that required drivers and front seat passengers of motor cars and light vans to wear seat belts. This requirement came into force on 1 February 1983 and was scheduled to run for a trial period of three years. Britain was relatively late in taking this step, most other developed countries having already done so.

At the end of the trial period a number of studies were carried out on behalf of the government and all agreed that the seat belt law had reduced the expected number of deaths and serious injuries on the road. Others, however, came to the opposite conclusion. Adams[7] sets out the position of the dissidents.

Three years is, of course, much too short a period for any degree of certainty about fatality rate trends. In Fig. 2.8, data for ten years before

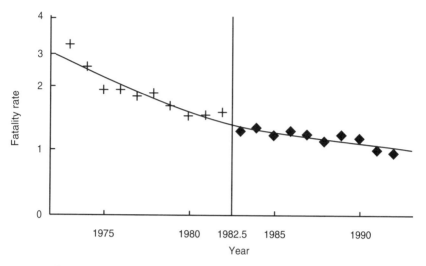

2.8 Annual fatality rate of motor car occupants per 10000 motor cars due to accidents on British roads, showing the effect of compulsory wearing of seat belts, 1973–92. +, 1973–83, annual decrement 5.2%; ◆, 1983–92, annual decrement 2.9%.

1983 and ten years afterwards are plotted together with their trend curves. These data are for annual deaths of motor car occupants per 10000 registered motor cars. Now there is no doubt about the fact that wearing a seat belt reduces the risk of death caused by a road accident. Numerous tests with dummies have demonstrated that, other things being equal, this is the case. There should, therefore, have been a discontinuity in the trend curves before and after 1983, that for the later period being displaced downwards by an amount corresponding to the extra safety afforded by the seat belts. This did not happen; the two trend curves meld together quite smoothly. Moreover, the relevant gradient post-1983 is over 40% lower than that before 1983. Thus, the compulsory wearing of seat belts, far from increasing the safety of motor car drivers and passengers, has had the opposite effect.

Adams,[7] who came to the same conclusion, suggests that drivers compensate for the extra safety afforded by the seat belt by taking greater chances, such that the overall risk remained the same. The smooth junction of the trend curves shown in Fig. 2.8 is consistent with this view, as is the lower annual decrement for the post-1983 period. It may further be surmised that if motor car drivers are behaving more recklessly, then pedestrian casualties should have increased in 1983. Figure 2.9 shows that

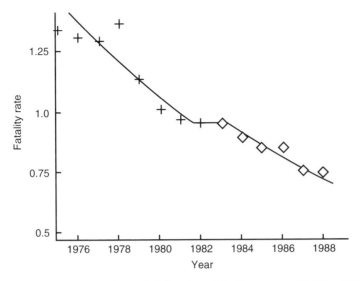

2.9 Effect of the 1983 seat belt law. Annual fatality rate per 10000 vehicles for pedestrians on British roads between 1971 and 1995 (period shown is 1975–88).

this was indeed the case and that the trend curve was displaced, but upwards instead of downwards.

It must not be supposed that such behaviour implies a negative attitude on the part of motor car drivers. In the year before the wearing of seat belts became compulsory, they were used by about 40% of drivers. After 1983 usage went up to 90% and has remained so. This represents a high degree of compliance, an acceptance of seat belts as necessary by the majority of drivers. Increased risk-taking, by contrast, was a subconscious reaction; motorists were quite unaware of the fact that they were killing pedestrians at a higher rate.

The efficacy of road safety legislation

It would appear, from the evidence presented above, that seat belt compulsion had a negative effect on safety. However, a plot of fatality rates of all road users for the decades before and after 1983 indicates no significant change in the relative gradients of the two trend curves, nor is there any discontinuity between them. The seat belt law therefore had no measurable effect on road safety. It has, however, provided a useful test case. No other piece of legislation has changed the behaviour of a large group of road users overnight. It could well be supposed that if the seat belt law was ineffective, then other road safety legislation is unlikely to succeed.

In Britain, major laws aimed at improving road safety (including the 1967 Breathalyser Act) came into force in the latter part of the twentieth century. Such measures should have resulted in an increase in the annual decrement in the road accident fatality rate. In fact this did not happen. For the period 1934–66 prior to the Breathalyser Act (ignoring the war years) the annual decrement was 5.04%, whilst that for 1967–2001 was 4.77%. The difference between these figures is not significant, but clearly there has been no measureable improvement. The road safety laws have indeed failed.

This is to be expected. Data presented here are consistent with the model proposed in Chapter 1, whereby the exponential fall in fatality is the result of the development of collective skills. This is a process that involves interactions between millions of individual human beings and is subconscious in character. Attempts to intervene in this process by arbitrary coercive means has (fortunately) very little chance of success.

The failure of punitive legal enactments to improve road safety may be contrasted with the success of successive generations of drivers in Britain. They have reduced the annual fatality rate per 10 000 vehicles from just over 30 in 1934 to 1.2 in the year 2000.

One of the problems that afflicts road safety (and which is also prevalent elsewhere) is that of partial statistics. From time to time it is found that applying a particular restriction in one location causes a reduction of road deaths in that location and it is argued that the use of this restriction nationwide would proportionally reduce the fatality rate. This argument assumes implicitly that human beings and human populations behave in the same way as inanimate matter. The evidence presented in this book (and, indeed, common sense) would gainsay any such notion. Partial statistics for a particular location are relevant only to that location. Road safety must be judged on the basis of national figures.

British railways

Figure 2.10 is a plot of the annual number of persons killed on British railways during successive five-year periods between 1900 and 1990. The figures are for the accidental deaths of passengers, staff, trespassers and others, such as pedestrians on level crossings; suicides are excluded. No attempt has been made to establish a rate because of the disparate nature of those concerned. Railway activity and usage may be measured by numbers of journeys undertaken. Surprisingly, this varied only marginally

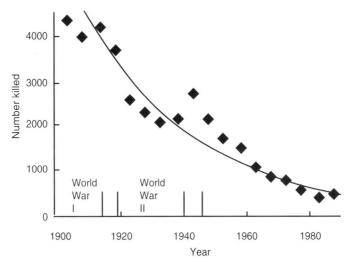

2.10 Number of persons killed annually on British railways, 1900–90. Data points represent five-year averages, plotted at the median of the five-year period. Annual decrement 2.7%, relative standard deviation 0.22.

during the twentieth century. Staff numbers, on the other hand, decreased to a considerable extent.

The plot shows a relatively wide scatter and two peaks corresponding to the two world wars. Otherwise there is a normal exponential fall. Passenger deaths due to train accidents do not fall in a regular fashion and are considered in the second part of this chapter.

Mortality from all causes

The mortality rates to be considered here are mainly those for England and Wales. These deaths are representative of a high proportion of the population of Britain. They are also likely to be similar to those for other Western European countries.

Arguments in favour of including all-cause mortality in this book are as follows:

1   The form taken by plots of mortality versus time for each individual age group is similar to that for most accident mortality data. There is an initial period where the trend is linear. Then at some point there is a switch to an exponentially falling rate with a more-or-less constant proportional gradient.

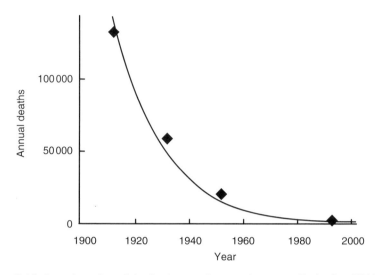

2.11 Annual number of deaths due to infectious diseases in England and Wales, 1911–91. The data points are plotted at 20-year intervals, starting at 1911. Annual decrement 5.2%.

2   The initial period of exponential fall is associated with a sharp reduction in the incidence of premature death due to infectious diseases such as cholera, typhus and tuberculosis of the lung.

3   Such deaths are due to the **accident of infection**. All-cause mortality could therefore be regarded as accident mortality in which the cause of death is biological instead of physical.

Figure 2.11 plots the annual number of deaths from infectious diseases in England and Wales during the period 1911–91. By 1970 the annual number of such deaths had been reduced by about 200 000. This number is similar to that which may be calculated from the known reduction in mortality rate assuming that population numbers remained constant. Thus there is numerical justification for propositions (2) and (3). Numbers aside, the conquest of infectious disease in developed countries is one of the greatest achievements of the twentieth century and one whose public recognition is long overdue.

A particular benefit of this change has been the reduction in infant mortality. The relevant figures for England and Wales, which date back to 1841, are plotted in Fig. 2.12. This indicates a modest linear fall in infant mortality rate of 0.06% annually, a switch to an exponential fall between 1895 and 1900 and a subsequent annual decrement of 3.47%.

Plots of mortality rate against time for other age groups take a similar form. However, the date of the switch to an exponential fall varies; for

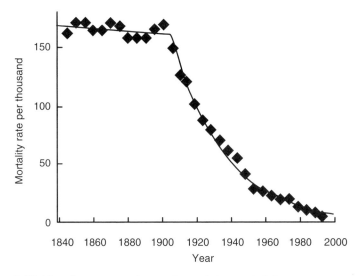

2.12 Mortality rate per thousand population: male infants up to one year of age, England and Wales, 1841–1995. Annual decrement, 1901–95, 3.47%.

children and young adults it occurred between 1860 and 1865, but the date becomes progressively later with increasing age. Infants were the latest to change, between 1895 and 1900.

The annual decrement in the mortality rate also varies with age. It is a maximum for infants, falling with increasing age, but with a slight hump at ages 35–45. Figure 2.13 shows mortality rates in England and Wales for the age group 65–74 between 1841 and 1995. The change to an exponential fall took place between 1891 and 1895 and the annual decrement after this time was 0.77%. Mortality rate plots for persons over 75 show a more gradual development of the falling rate.

It would seem, therefore, that all-cause mortality may indeed be regarded as the result of a biological accident, such that the pattern of events should be similar to that for physical accidents. In particular, the fact that young men take greater risks than women of the same age should be reflected in mortality records.

This is indeed the case. Figure 2.14 plots the ratio between male and female mortality in England and Wales for the year 2000. The form of this plot is almost precisely similar to that for physical accidents as portrayed in Fig. 1.2. It is not easy to accept the notion that the risk of death from disease can be manipulated in the same way as accidental death, but the record clearly shows this to be the case. There is no element of suicide here: the higher fatality rate results from a different, subconsciously motivated behaviour.

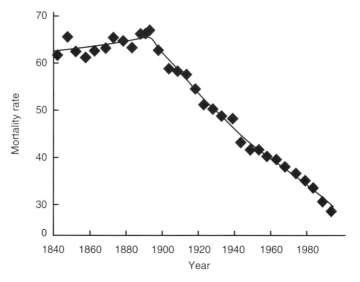

2.13 Mortality rate per thousand population for persons in the age group 65–74, England and Wales, 1841–1995. Annual decrement 0.77%.

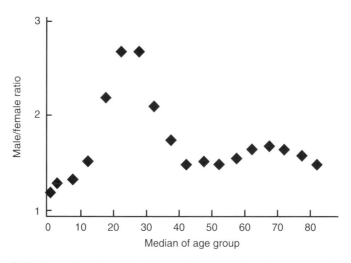

2.14 Ratio of male and female mortality rates dependent on age, England and Wales, 2000.

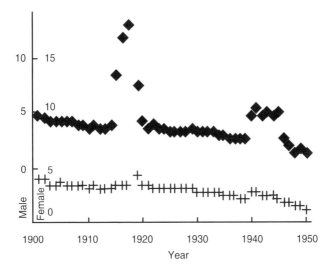

2.15 Mortality rate per thousand population for the 20–24 age group in England and Wales annually, 1900–50. The data point for 1918, when mortality rate was about 27, is not plotted. ◆, male; +, female. Annual decrement for both sexes is 1.7%. For clarity, the female curve has been displaced downwards. Note the different scales.

It was earlier surmised that the tendency for civilian accident mortality to increase during times of war was largely due to the behaviour of young men. Such is certainly the case for all-cause mortality. Figure 2.15 shows male and female mortality rates separately for the 20–24 age group in England and Wales for 1901–50. These rates relate to civilian deaths during wartime, not those of the armed forces. Charlton[8] suggests that the high male wartime rates were due to the enlistment of fit men into the armed forces, leaving a sickly remnant whose death rate was higher. However, suppose that all pre-war deaths occurred within the sickly portion of the age group. In wartime the mortality rate would go up, but number of deaths would be about the same; in fact they increased. Thus, for the 20–24 age group, numbers of deaths were: 1913, 5354; 1914, 5909; 1915, 7222; 1916, 7459; 1917, 7009; 1918, 13 520. All the war years show an increase (the very large number in 1918 was due to the influenza epidemic of that year). In 1920 and subsequently, death numbers returned to the pre-war level.

The increase in mortality rates amongst young men during wartime must therefore be put down to the human factor. Finding a more precise descriptive name for this phenomenon is difficult; nor is it at all obvious how the increase is accomplished. It is easy to understand how a higher level of risk can increase the probability of a physical accident, but not for contracting a fatal disease. However, the fact that mortality rates are falling in an orderly fashion implies that the population as a whole is in control of the risk of fatal infections. That being so, it is surely possible for part of the population to change the risk in the opposite sense.

Two other features of Fig. 2.15 deserve mention. First, assuming that the amount of the upward shift in mortality rate is a measure of the degree of enthusiasm for the war, then such enthusiasm was much less evident on the second occasion than on the first. This accords with recollection and other historical evidence; during the first part of the First World War the armed forces were manned by volunteers. During the Second World War, however, conscription was used from the start.

Second, women showed no enthusiasm for either war. The slight increase in female mortality during the 1939–45 War was almost certainly due to the aerial bombing of cities.

Figure 2.15 shows only a small difference between the peacetime mortality rates for males and females, in apparent contradiction to the large difference indicated by Fig. 2.14. In fact, this difference only appeared during the second half of the twentieth century. Perhaps the more sterile conditions prevailing during that period gave added scope to risky behaviour.

Mortality and medicine

The date when the exponential fall in mortality rates began – the early 1860s – may well provide a clue to the nature of this relationship. Pasteur began his work on fermentation in 1850. This led to an understanding that disease could be transmitted by living organisms. The next decade saw improvements in drinking water and sewage disposal in London and other cities. It has been shown earlier that technological change does not directly influence accident rates, but may provide the conditions under which the human population effects improvements. Thus, better sanitation and an understanding of the need for hygiene were probably essential elements in the development of skill in the avoidance of infection. 1860 is a credible date for such circumstances to arise.

So the ordered reduction in mortality rates resulted from a change in the behaviour of the population (in this instance of England and Wales) as a whole. As for other such falling rates, the associated learning process was subconscious. Medication played no part in these events since, at the time, no effective medicines were available. Doctors, however, played an essential part in providing an understanding of the nature of infective agents and in contributing to improvements in public hygiene.

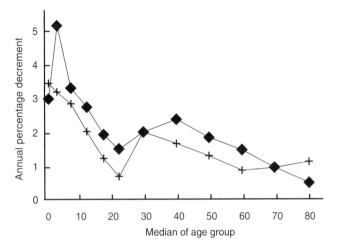

2.16 Annual percentage decrement trend curve for mortality rate versus time, females, England and Wales, ♦, 1901–50; +, 1951–2000. Average decrement, 1901–50, 2.24%; 1951–2000, 1.79%.

In developed countries effective medicines became generally available during the period following the Second World War. These, combined with developments in surgical techniques, led to a radical improvement in the effectiveness of medical care. These developments have greatly improved the quality of life for those suffering either physical or biological accidents and in many instances lives have been prolonged by medication or surgery. So it might reasonably be expected that the mortality rate would fall more rapidly during the second half of the twentieth century than it did during the years before 1950. In fact, this was not the case, at least in England and Wales. Figure 2.16 compares the annual decrement in fatality rate for females in these countries between 1901 and 1950 with those for 1950–2001. The comparison was restricted to females in order to eliminate distortions caused by war in the first period. However, a similar plot for persons (both sexes taken together) yields a very similar result. Thus, for most age groups, mortality rates declined more slowly during the second half of the twentieth century than they did during the first half. Only for the very young and the very old was there an increase. The average annual decrement (or relative gradient of the trend curve) for all groups fell by 20%.

In summary, plots of all-cause mortality rates for the various age groups in England and Wales are generally similar in form to those for mortality due to physical accidents. There is an initial period during which data follow a linear trend which is level or decreases slightly. Then, in the early 1860s, there was, for most age groups, a switch to an exponentially falling trend, which has continued subsequently. The plot for older persons up to age 75 was similar in form to those for young age groups, but the exponential fall was initiated later and the annual decrement is lower. It is concluded that all-cause mortality may be interpreted as being due to a biological accident, that of infection by a fatal disorder. Thus, the exponential fall in mortality rates is the result of the development of collective skills in avoiding infections. It is not surprising, then, that all-cause mortality records have characteristics similar to those of the 'normal' type of physical accident. Notably such systems are self-regulating and are unresponsive to attempts by outside organisations to change their course. In particular, the formation of the National Health Service in Britain and the development of effective medicines did not cause mortality rates in England and Wales to diminish any faster than before. Good medical practice can improve the quality of life, but it is the population at large that determines the rate at which we die.

Exceptions

Motorcycles

Most people would agree with the proposition that a motorcycle is less safe than a four-wheeled vehicle. The rider is completely exposed. In the event of a collision he or she is likely to be thrown on to the road, possibly in front of oncoming traffic. But facts do not always conform to preconceptions. Figure 2.17 shows fatality rates per 10 000 motorcycles on British roads between 1930 and 1959. This is remarkably similar to that for all vehicles (Fig. 2.6). There is an early period up to 1934 when the trend was linear and rising. Then in 1934 there was a switch to an exponentially falling rate, interrupted during the 1939–45 War by an abrupt upsurge. The date of the switch (1934) is the same for both plots and the fatality rate at that time was also the same, about 30 deaths per year per 10 000 vehicles.

In the early days the British motorcycle was the poor man's motor car and the riders were able to compensate for the inherent disadvantages of a two-wheeled vehicle to such a degree that the fatality record matched that for traffic generally.

The match was not quite perfect, however. The annual decrement in the fatality rate for motorcycles between 1934 and 1959 was 4.4%, whilst that for all vehicles for the same period was 5.6%. Now it was seen earlier that greater risk-taking on the part of motor car drivers after the seat belt law resulted in a reduction in the annual decrement. It is possible, in the case of motorcycles, that a non-comforming minority of riders affected the fatality rate and its decrement.

However this may be, the situation changed in the early 1960s when British motorcycling became a hazardous sport. Figure 2.18 plots annual

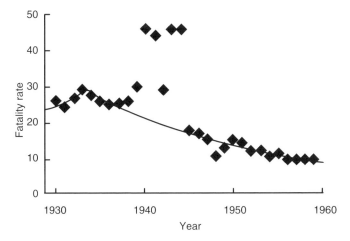

2.17 Annual fatality rate for motorcyclists per 10000 registered motorcycles on British roads, 1930–59. Annual decrement for the period 1934–59 (ignoring the war years) 4.4%.

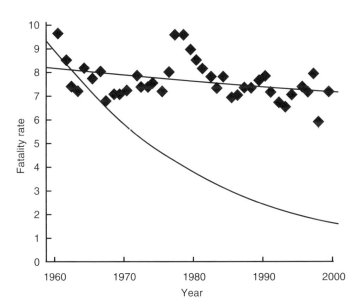

2.18 Fatality rate per 10000 motorcycles for motorcycle riders on British roads, 1960–2000. No significant trend. The lower line is an extrapolation of the trend curve for 1934–59.

fatality rates for motorcycle riders from 1960 to 2000. There is much scatter of data, but the trend is linear and the average rate almost constant. It would seem that after 1960 the risk-taking minority became dominant, maintaining the risk as closely as possible at the 1960 level. A plot of annual deaths and motorcycle numbers shows that these two quantities follow a very similar course, suggesting that the fatality risk may have been more constant than Fig. 2.18 would suggest.

Also shown in Fig. 2.18 is an extrapolation of the trend curve for the 1934–59 period. The gap between this curve and the upper horizontal line represents several thousand lives unnecessarily lost, together with a very much greater number of injuries.

Motorcycle sport came into being as a result of the general loosening of social discipline that occurred during the 1960s. The cost of this laxity is a heavy one.

Passengers on British railways

It was recorded in the first part of this chapter that the number of persons (including passengers, staff and others) killed on British railways showed a normal trend, that is to say, they diminished exponentially with time. In the case of passengers killed in train accidents, however, the historical record is less simple.

On the day that the world's first regular service on a dedicated track was inaugurated, a passenger was killed (the circumstances are described in Chapter 3). Passenger losses in train accidents are of special concern. Usually numbers are small, but from time to time there is a major incident which attracts wide publicity. British railways' records of such losses date back to 1875. Figures for numbers of journeys are also available, enabling a rate to be established.

Figure 2.19 shows the number of passengers killed in train accidents per billion journeys from 1875 to 2002. The data plotted are ten-year averages except for the last period, which is the average for 1995–2002. A ten-year period was chosen firstly because early figures are ten-year averages, secondly because year-to-year variations are large and thirdly to eliminate zeros whilst still taking account of them.

Figure 2.19 displays the result. There was an exponential fall from 1875 to 1920, then a linear increase to a peak in the early 1950s, followed by a further exponential fall to 2002. The hidden clock is operating here, because the second exponential trend curve falls to a level close to the extrapolation of the first.

It would seem that a proportion of the railway workforce became disaffected during the 1920s and began to operate the system in an unsafe

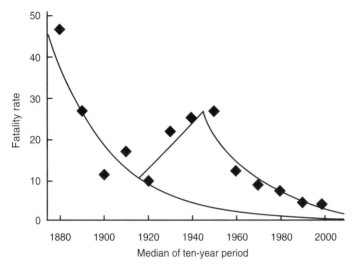

2.19 Annual passenger fatality rate per billion journeys due to train accidents on British railways, 1875–2002. Data points represent ten-year averages.

manner, culminating in the Harrow and Wealdstone double collision in 1952, where 112 people were killed. Following this incident there was a change in behaviour and passenger safety improved rapidly to a level that could be regarded as reasonable. The hidden clock was, of course, that proportion of the workforce that continued to operate normally. The return to acceptable safety operating levels has not been accompanied by any significant improvement in efficiency. In the early twenty-first century the system is characterised by poor timekeeping, train cancellations, and so on. Safety and efficiency do not necessarily march together.

The oil industry

It is exceptional, when analysing the loss and fatality record of the oil industry to come across the 'normal' case of an exponentially falling rate. Operators in this industry come from a great variety of countries, but the technology is predominantly American and practice is remarkably uniform. So, too, is the attitude towards work: with a few exceptions it is very positive. Thus, if there is a lack of safety in any area it is more likely to be due to an excess of zeal rather than otherwise.

Oil and gas operators may be considered under three headings: exploration, production and processing. These phases are described in Chapter 5. For the casualty record, the first two will be taken together. The interest here is for offshore exploration and production, for which good data are available.

Exploration and production

The first step in exploration is to identify an area where oil bearing strata may be present. The second is to drill a test well. This operation is carried out using a mobile offshore unit. Once a potentially productive area has been found, the mobile unit is replaced by a stationary platform, from which production wells are drilled.

There are various sources of information concerning offshore casualties, but the most comprehensive is the worldwide offshore accident databank,[9] which is maintained by Det Norsk Veritas in Oslo, Norway.

Figure 2.20 plots the annual percentage loss of mobile offshore units during the period 1970–97. There is a substantial reduction in the loss rate during this period, but instead of falling continuously it does so stepwise and on either side of the step the trend is linear and more or less flat. It is instructive to compare these losses with those of commercial shipping. For the period prior to the stepwise fall, 1970–90, the average losses were off-shore units 1.1%; ships 0.5%, whilst after the step change, 1991–97, they were 0.21% for offshore and 0.28% for ships. The comparison is not unreasonable. Many offshore mobile units are modified barge-like vessels,

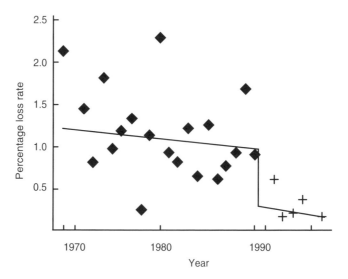

2.20 Annual percentage loss of mobile units off-shore worldwide, 1970–97.[9]
◆, 1970–90; +, 1991–97.

but some are converted oil tankers. They operate on the continental shelf, not too far from land, but the weather can be just as severe as in deep water. In any event, there seems to be little difference in the later loss rates.

Figure 2.21 shows the fatality rate for offshore mobile units, expressed here as the annual number of deaths per 100 operating units. As would be expected, the trend is similar to that for the unit losses except that fatality rates rose prior to 1990. Fatality rates for fixed units show a very similar pattern, but some large individual losses (due to the *Piper Alpha* catastrophe, for example) make it difficult to establish the trend with reasonable certainty. Losses of fixed units are too small to justify statistical analysis.

Where the casualty rate falls exponentially with time, the relevant activity has a self-regulating character and is unresponsive to external events other than a world war. In the present instance, however, such may not be the case and it is tempting to look for the circumstance that might have triggered the precipitous fall in 1990. A possible candidate is the economic recession that affected a number of developed countries at that time. However, this recession had remarkably little effect on world crude oil production. Between 1987 and 1996 oil output increased exponentially, with an increment of 1.3% annually. Between 1990 and 1991 there was a fall in output of 0.6%, but this was well within the normal scatter band.

Alternatively, it is possible that the discrepancy between the risk of operating mobile units and that of commercial shipping became untenable.

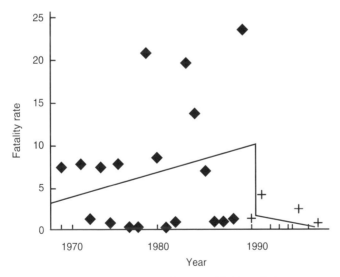

2.21 Annual fatality rate per 100 units. Mobile off-shore units, worldwide, 1970–97.[9]

In 1990 the offshore loss rate was 0.9% and that for shipping was 0.24%. In 1991 the offshore mobile loss rate fell to 0.21%. The numbers are consistent with this interpretation.

The one thing that is certain is that this rapid change could not come from any physical cause such as better weather or improved equipment. It must have been due to a change in human behaviour.

Hydrocarbon processing

The raw material for a large section of the chemical industry is either natural gas or a product obtained by refining crude oil. Oil refineries also produce the fuel for air, land and sea transport: aviation fuel, gasoline, diesel oil and heavy fuel oil. In the twenty-first century oil and gas produce a major part of the energy that is required for the well-being of the industrialised nations.

The oil refinery, which is a key element in this process, handles an inflammable and sometimes explosive substance, such that accidents during operation of the plant can lead to much physical damage and financial loss. The fatality risk to human operators however is small; they are not numerous and the control room can be well protected. The accident rate may best be estimated from the resultant financial losses. The relevant data have been collected and published for numbers of years by an insurance broker, Marsh & McLennan of Chicago.[10] This survey records the 100 largest financial losses that occurred during the previous 30 years and covers oil refineries, gas treatment plant, petrochemical and power industry equipment. The data is selective in that smaller losses below about ten million dollars are not included. It constitutes, nevertheless, a large and representative sample. Losses are quoted in US dollars at constant prices.

Figure 2.22 shows how such losses have changed during the period 1967–96. Up to the 1987–91 period there was a generally rising trend, but the next five-year period showed a sharp fall. Figures for the number of plants affected show a very similar pattern (Fig. 2.23).

These data are taken from a summary survey that is published every five years.[10] They cover all types of hydrocarbon processing plant, including petrochemicals. When the first edition of this book was written, only the rising part of these curves was extant. This was contrary to the general experience of accident rates. The present author, following the cause-and-effect theory, ascribed the rise to physical factors such as a concentration of assets on smaller sites, the increased incidence of vapour cloud explosions, and so forth. The original compiler of the survey provided similar explanations. These ideas, however, are quite incompatible with the fall that occurred in 1992–96, in spite of the continued presence of all the

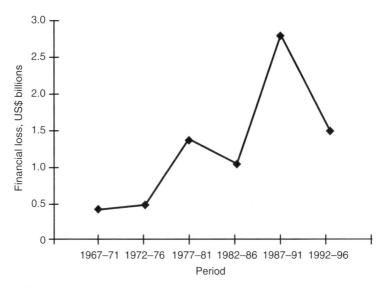

2.22 Capital cost of major accidents in hydrocarbon process plant, worldwide, 1967–96.

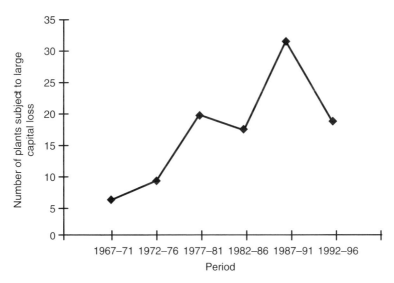

2.23 Number of hydrocarbon process plants subject to large capital loss worldwide, 1967–96.

physical factors. The fall must, indeed, have been due to a change in human behaviour.

In order to expand and update this information, annual data have been extracted for refineries only from the 2003 edition of the Marsh & McLennan survey. The loss figures have been divided by the nominal value of the crude oil produced worldwide.[11] The value of crude oil is taken as US$100 per metric ton. This provides a measure of the significance of the financial losses.

The results are plotted in Fig. 2.24. This shows a rising trend to a peak in 1992, then an 87% fall to a low value in 1993, followed by a further rise.

The Marsh & McLennan document includes a description of the events leading up to the losses recorded. In these there are a few cases of gross error; for the most part, a process upset occurred and the operators were unable to correct it. Nevertheless, even with computer-assisted controls, it is possible to operate a unit up to the limit of its capacity, and thereby to increase the risk of a failure. The sudden drop in the loss rate in 1992 suggests a rather sudden return to more conservative practices. The plot also suggests that history might repeat itself in a few years' time.

The fall in offshore mobile unit losses occurred in 1990. It is possible that these two activities shared a common sense of optimism with the population in some developed countries and that the bubble burst in successive stages: the London Stock Market in 1987, the British economy

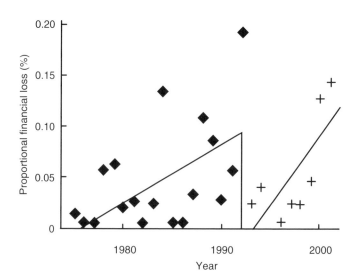

2.24 Financial loss due to accidents during operation of oil refineries world-wide 1975–2001, expressed as a percentage of the nominal value of crude oil produced. ◆, 1975–92; +, 1993–2001. The peak figure is 0.19% for 1992.

in 1989, followed by the sudden fall in offshore mobile unit fatalities and of financial loss due to oil refinery accidents.

However, the peak financial loss due to accidents in oil refineries cost only about 0.2% of the value of the oil that they processed. This is an affordable figure and may well be less than other losses due to theft, piracy, spillage and so forth.

Changing human behaviour

In those activities where casualty rates are falling exponentially, any attempt to interfere with the process would be most unwise. There are, however, exceptional cases where attempts have been made to improve safety by modifying the behaviour of the people concerned.

One such case was in engineering construction. This activity was not recorded as an exception in the previous section of this chapter because in the late 1990s fatality rates started to decrease. In earlier times however (as noted in previous editions of this book) fatality rates in construction work were about ten times that for manufacturing industry and were not falling. The MW Kellogg Company, Houston-based chemical engineers, took a special interest in this problem and set up a safety campaign on their own worldwide construction sites. Every conceivable step was taken but most especially the support of the workforce and the trades unions was obtained. Within a period of two years the fatality rate fell to a level close to that for factories. Further reductions however proved to be difficult.

Professor Robertson, a psychologist at the University of Manchester Institute of Science and Technology, carried out similar work on engineering construction sites in north-west England, and likewise succeeded in reducing accidents. The method was first to identify locations with a safety risk, then to set targets for their improvement (for example, ensuring that all scaffolding platforms were fully boarded) and to give periodical reports of progress to the workers on site. In the USA, psychologists have applied such techniques to reduce fatalities and injuries in factories.

Such activities are necessarily on a relatively small scale and would not be reflected in industry-wide statistics. They could, however, be of value in locations where casualty rates are above the norm.

There is no record of the control of accident rates on a large scale, such as for particular industries or modes of transport. Earlier in this chapter the futility of government legislation and punitive action in the case of British manufacturing industry and of road transport was noted. Large populations are self-regulating in such matters.

National productivity and accident rates

National productivity, or national output per head, or per capita gross domestic product, is the value of all national products divided by the population number. In this book the gross domestic product is expressed at constant prices; that is to say, values are adjusted to compensate for monetary inflation.

A general relationship between national productivity and fatal accident rates was established in Chapter 1. This being the case, it seems reasonable to suppose that where there is a change in the national mood, say from optimistic recklessness to pessimistic caution, then both productivity and accident rates would be affected.

Figure 2.25 illustrates such a case. The early 1990s saw major downturns in productive activity in a number of developed countries. In the UK the depression occurred in 1989. To obtain Fig. 2.25(a) the trend curve for per capita gross domestic product at constant prices for the period 1950–2000[12] was established, and the percentage deviation from this curve plotted for 1987–96. A similar procedure was adopted for the fatality rate in accidents on British roads, the result of which is shown in Fig. 2.25(b).

These two figures are remarkably similar. Both show a strong rising trend, followed by a sudden collapse, then a further rising trend. The pattern of events was similar to that of financial loss due to accidents in oil refineries, shown in Fig. 2.24, which was also tentatively linked to economic recession. So it would seem that the association between accident rates and economic trends may apply to the 'boom and bust' cycle. The other major perturbation to national productivity in Britain during the twentieth century occurred as a result of the two world wars.

Figure 2.26 shows percentage deviation from the 1900–49 trend curve for the period 1938–46. The trend curve was calculated from data listed by Feinstein[13] after eliminating wartime data. A similar upsurge occurred during the First World War, but it was not quite so high. These increases were wholly or partially due to longer hours of work; this implies an element of patriotic zeal. The same factor is represented in Fig. 2.27, which shows (a) all-cause mortality rate for civilian males in the 20–24 age group and (b) fatality rates in road accidents. The cause-and-effect theory would ascribe the increased mortality amongst young men to the creaming-off by conscription of the fit ones. However, conscription did not stop in 1946, but continued for some years, although the higher mortality rate returned to normal when hostilities ceased.

In all these comparisons the percentage increase of fatality rates is much higher than that of productivity. This is hardly surprising: recklessness knows no bounds, but the production of nuts and bolts most certainly does.

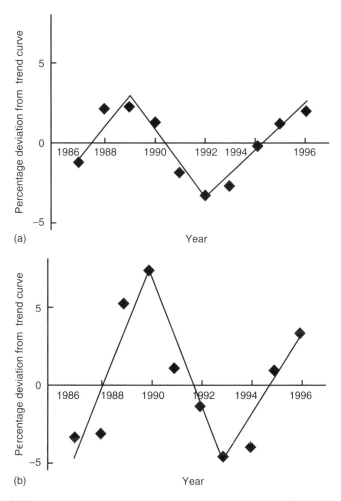

2.25 Percentage deviation from trend curve during the 1989 economic recession, Britain: (a) per capita gross domestic product; (b) fatality rate in road accidents.

Conclusions

1   There is a general tendency for accident mortality rates, and for mortality rates from all causes, to decrease with the passage of time. Where records extend sufficiently far back, there is an initial phase during which the trend is linear and may be level, falling or (exceptionally) rising. Then, in most industries and modes of transport there is a switch to an exponential fall. This condition, which became the norm during the twentieth century, is considered to be the result

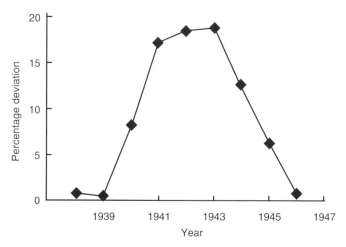

2.26 Per capita gross domestic product, Britain. Percentage deviation from the 1900–49 trend curve during the Second World War.

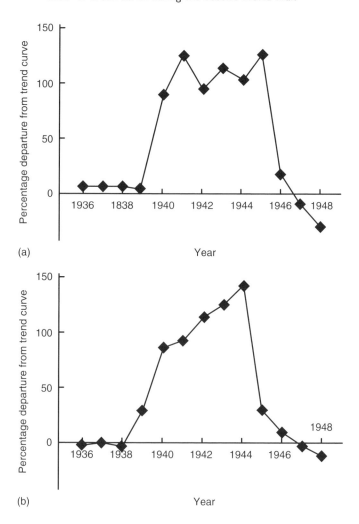

of a subconscious development of collective skill, such that the population concerned becomes more adept at avoiding fatal accidents and fatal infections.

2   A simple mathematical model for the exponential fall appears to represent most data adequately. Such developments are associated with increases in national productivity, which is similarly the result of the subconscious development of collective skills, and increases exponentially with time.

3   Technological developments and other consciously directed improvements are permissive factors. They do not directly influence safety, but provide a framework within which the human population can make progress. Technology provides the opportunity, but the human factor determines the rapidity with which casualty rates diminish.

4   In most instances it is impossible to relate the initiation of the exponential fall in casualty rates to any particular event or circumstance. Nor is the population concerned consciously aware of the change. It seems likely, however, that a sufficiently high level of technological development is an essential factor.

5   Once the exponential fall in casualty rate has been established the process is self-regulating and the proportional gradient of the trend curve that best represents the data is more or less constant. External events, other than major wars, do not directly affect the trend in accident rates. In particular, attempts by government to influence such trends by legislation and punitive action are at best ineffectual and may be counter-productive.

6   Fatality rates due to accident and disease are not uniform with respect to sex and age. For females such rates increase steadily with increasing age. For males the rates tend to increase with age to a maximum around the 20–24 age group, then decrease, and later increase again. These discrepancies were more pronounced during the two world wars.

7   These conclusions apply both to fatalities due to physical accidents and those due to all causes. Plots of all-cause mortality rates against time during the twentieth century follow the same type of exponential fall as physical accidents, and conform to similar general rules.

2.27 Percentage departure from trend curve during the Second World War. (a) All-cause mortality rate for civilian males in the 20–24 age group, England and Wales, 1936–48. (b) Fatality rate in road accidents, civilians in Britain, 1936–48.

Note

Subconscious learning, although not a matter of everyday conversation, is nevertheless one of common experience. Learning to talk and learning to walk are examples, all except a few unfortunate individuals having passed through these processes. Such instances however concern individuals, whereas in the present context we are dealing with subconscious collective learning, where individuals learn by example from other members of the population. It is possible that especially skilled persons provide leadership in the progressive development that has been recorded here.

The fact that such developments occur below the level of consciousness makes their analysis rather difficult. However, it is clear that interactions between large numbers of individuals are an essential feature of the process. It has been proposed that the observed fall in casualty rates is the result of a positive attitude towards improvement on the part of the population concerned. It may further be argued that where such a positive attitude exists, the proportional scatter of the data relative to the trend curve should be reduced. In Appendix 1, a comparison is made with a system where interactions are purely physical, and it is found that in the human case, where there is an exponential fall in casualty rates, the scatter of data is indeed reduced. There is some evidence, therefore, for the rather primitive model of collective learning that is presented here.

References

1. The Office for National Statistics, *Road Accidents Great Britain*, published annually by HM Stationery Office, London.
2. Health and Safety Executive, 'Numbers of persons killed in industrial accidents, 1880–1968'. *Historical Injury Data*.
3. Department of Employment, *British Labour Statistics*, HM Stationery Office, London, 1971.
4. Health and Safety Executive, *Fatal Injury Rates*, 1981–2000.
5. Department of Employment and Productivity, *British Labour Statistics*, HM Stationery Office, London, 1971.
6. *Statistical Summary of Commercial Jet Aircraft Accidents, Worldwide Operations*, Boeing Commercial Aircraft Group, Seattle, USA (published annually).
7. Adams, J. 'Smeed's Law, seat belts, and the Emperor's new clothers', *Human Behaviour and Traffic Safety*, General Motors, Detroit, 1986.
8. Charlton, J. *The Health of Adult Britain 1841 to 1994*, Office for National Statistics, London.
9. Det Norsk Veritas, *Worldwide Offshore Accident Databank*, 1998 edition, Oslo, Norway. Publication ceased in 1998 but the database is being retained.
10. Marsh & McLennan, *Large property damage losses in the hydrocarbon–chemical industry*, 20th Edn., Chicago, 2003.

11. British Petroleum, *BP Statistical Review of World Energy* (published annually).
12. Office for National Statistics, *United Kingdom National Accounts – the Blue Book*, 2004.
13. Feinstein, C.H. *National Income, Expenditure and Output of the United Kingdom 1855 to 1965*, Cambridge University Press, 1972.

CHAPTER 3

Supercatastrophes

The large-scale accidents described in this chapter cannot be treated statistically in the way that fatality and loss rates have been dealt with in earlier chapters. There are however some common features of human behaviour in maritime accidents that are noted under the heading 'Comment' at the end of this chapter.

Shipping accidents

The Titanic

The doomed ship has always figured largely in the literature of human disaster. William Rees-Mogg, with greater concern for dramatic effect than for dull reality, put it thus:

> This sinking of the *Titanic* in 1912 is one of the most popular metaphors for the condition of mankind. The reckless speed, the competition for the Blue Riband of the Atlantic, the wealth and luxury of the First Class, the cramped poverty of the steerage, the foolishness of those who believed the ship unsinkable, the negligence of the captain, the arrogance of mankind in the face of nature – all make the story a parable for today.[1]

Well said, but like other purveyors of *Titanic* myths, Rees-Mogg was wrong on almost every count. It was said that the excessive speed was due to an intention to make the fastest transatlantic crossing and capture the Blue Riband. But this was a physical impossibility; the rival Cunard ships had more power and less weight. The White Star Line, which owned the *Titanic*, aimed to compete in size and luxury, not in speed. Another theory is that there was a fire in one of the bunkers and the captain was anxious to reach New York before it burst into flames. The tale has no end.

Design features

To forget the myths for the moment, the actuality began in the shipyards of Harland and Wolff in Belfast during the early years of the twentieth century. The *Titanic* (shown in section in Fig. 3.1) was one of three sister ships, the other two being the *Olympic* and the *Britannic*. They were built to include the latest available technology. Originally it was intended that they should be twin-screw ships driven by reciprocating engines, but at a later stage a third screw was added, driven by a steam turbine. There was a double bottom, but the feature that made headlines was that the hull was divided into watertight compartments. At the base of each bulkhead that formed a compartment was a door, normally held up by an electromagnet.

These doors were operated from the bridge: in an emergency an alarm would sound, and after an interval of time long enough to allow the crew to escape, the door came down. Those who failed to get through the doors in time would escape by ladders. The ships were designed to remain afloat with two compartments flooded. It may have been foolish to think that the *Titanic* was unsinkable, but it was in fact reasonably secure against most of the likely hazards. At the present time loss due to a grazing collision (contact) is relatively rare, amounting to about 4% of the total, and there is no reason to believe that matters were different in the days of the *Titanic*. Most other accidents would have flooded one, or at most two, of the compartments, so it could be argued that the ship was about 95% unsinkable.

When it was launched on 31 May 1911 the *Titanic* was the largest ship in the world, with a length of 825.5 ft and 92.5 ft across the beam. The ship is shown at berth in Fig. 3.2 and the opulence of the First Class section illustrated in Fig. 3.3. The displacement was 46 382 tons, compared with an average (for 1910) of about 1400 tons. After being fitted out and undergoing sea trials, the *Titanic* left Southampton to start her maiden voyage on 10 April 1912 with 922 passengers on board. While she was leaving, there was a near-collision with a moored vessel. When two ships pass at close quarters the water between them flows at an increased speed, with a corresponding fall in pressure. As a result, the ships move towards each other. This happened in the case of the *Titanic*. Disaster was only averted by prompt action on the part of the master, Captain Smith, and by the accompanying tugboats.

Later the same day she called at Cherbourg and took on 274 more passengers. On the following day she stopped at the Irish port of Queenstown and took on a further 120 people, mostly Irish emigrants to the United States. The *Titanic* finally set off across the Atlantic on 11 April with a complement of 2228 passengers and crew. The UK Board of Trade regulations required that ships with a displacement of over 10 000 tons should carry 16 lifeboats. The *Titanic* carried, in addition to the required number, four collapsible boats, giving a total capacity of 1178 persons, about half the number on board and about one-third of the maximum

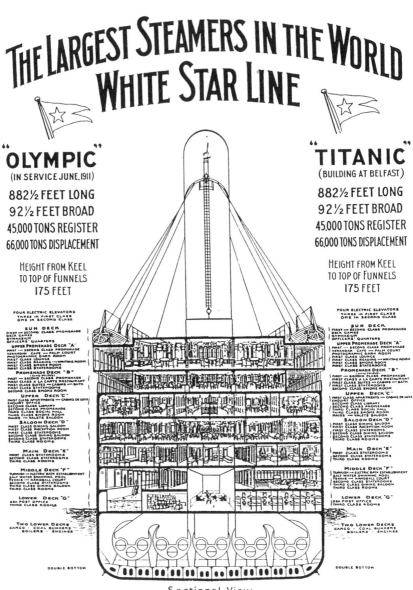

THE LARGEST STEAMERS IN THE WORLD
WHITE STAR LINE

"OLYMPIC"
(IN SERVICE JUNE, 1911)

882½ FEET LONG
92½ FEET BROAD
45,000 TONS REGISTER
66,000 TONS DISPLACEMENT

HEIGHT FROM KEEL
TO TOP OF FUNNELS
175 FEET

"TITANIC"
(BUILDING AT BELFAST)

882½ FEET LONG
92½ FEET BROAD
45,000 TONS REGISTER
66,000 TONS DISPLACEMENT

HEIGHT FROM KEEL
TO TOP OF FUNNELS
175 FEET

Sectional View
(AMIDSHIP)
THE TRIPLE SCREW SEA GIANTS
"OLYMPIC" ☆ "TITANIC"

3.1 The White Star Line, based in Liverpool, was owned by J P Morgan, the American financier and railroad millionaire, at the time when the *Titanic* sank.

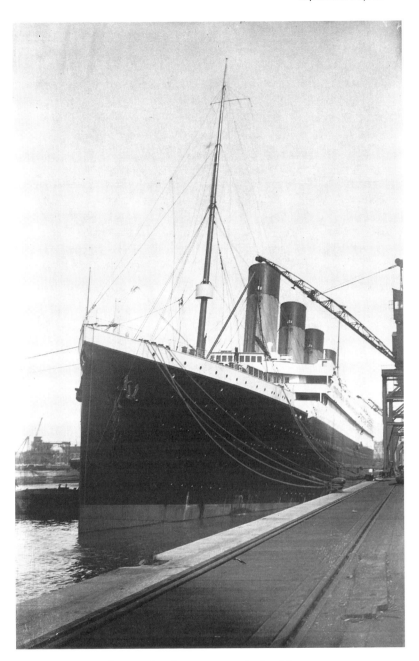

3.2 The *Titanic* at berth, just prior to its fateful voyage.

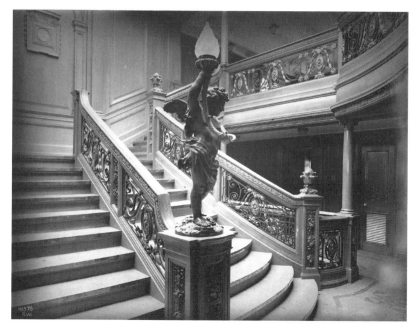

3.3 '. . . the wealth and luxury of the First Class . . .' – the grand staircase of the sister ship *Olympic*. The staircase of the *Titanic* was similar and may be seen today in ghostly video pictures taken inside the wreck.

complement of 3300. By contrast, regulations at that time specified that cargo ships should carry lifeboats with a capacity of twice the ship's complement, it being argued that when a ship was sinking, it could well list in such a way that only half the lifeboats could be launched.

The sinking

On the night of 14/15 April the ship was steaming at full speed, about 22 knots. The weather was still and frosty, cloudless but with no moon, and the sea was dead calm. There had been warnings of ice ahead by wireless from other ships. The most recent call was from the *Californian*, a British ship located a few miles away, which was stationary because of field ice in the vicinity. At the same time the radio operator of the *Titanic* was passing messages from the passengers to US destinations and the backlog was such that he declined to accept the call. Shortly after this, the radio operator on the *Californian* finished his watch and went below. A short time later still, the *Titanic* struck an iceberg and sank.

It was by no means unusual to encounter icebergs in the North Atlantic in April, but in 1912 the ice had drifted further south than usual. The normal precaution against colliding with an iceberg at night was to extinguish or mask lights forward of the bridge and post lookouts. This was done on the *Titanic*, with two men aloft and two officers on the bridge. It was customary to keep watch by naked eye; binoculars or telescopes restrict the field of view. All should have been well, but when the iceberg was sighted, it was only about a quarter of a mile ahead. The officer of the watch immediately ordered full astern and put the helm hard over. The distance was too short, however, and the ship received a series of glancing blows over a length of about 250 ft. These caused plating to buckle and rivets to shear or fail in tension, cracking the caulking. Water then flooded into five, possibly six, of the forward compartments.

The impact occurred at 11.40 pm and some time elapsed before the captain gave the order to man the lifeboats. Women and children were to board first, but it proved difficult to persuade married women to leave their husbands behind. In the steerage particularly, passengers were reluctant to leave their belongings (mostly the only things they possessed), particularly as the stern portion of the ship was dry. Eventually the 16 boats and one collapsible were launched and other collapsibles pitched into the sea.

Throughout this period the crew behaved in exemplary fashion, attending to their duties to the end. The engine-room staff maintained power and the lights shone brilliantly until just before the final plunge; none of these men survived. Only one of the senior officers was saved; this was Second Officer C H Lightoller. He walked down the sloping deck into the sea, after freeing the last of the collapsible boats. After being pulled down he was blown to the surface by a sudden uprush of water, and then managed to scramble on to an upturned collapsible. Captain Smith remained on deck directing operations until it was clear that no more could be done; he then walked forward calmly to take his place on the bridge. The ship went down at 2.20 am with the loss of over 1500 lives.

The rescue

Several ships picked up the wireless distress signal CQD, the nearest of which was the *Carpathia*, about 30 miles distant. All these ships steamed at full speed towards the wreck until the *Carpathia* signalled her arrival. Some put an extra watch in the stokehold in order to find a little more speed. The *Carpathia* picked up the survivors. According to the master of the *Carpathia* these numbered 705, but the purser later added six more making a total of 711. This figure was adopted officially, but the captain subsequently maintained that his original number was correct.

The enigmatic feature of this period is the role of the *Californian*. There was no radio operator on duty, so the distress calls on the wireless were not heard. As well as radio signals, the crew of the *Titanic* also indicated their situation by sending up distress rockets. Officers on board the *Californian* saw the flashes from these rockets, but were uncertain about their significance. They tried to communicate with the unknown vessel by Morse lamp but without success. After a time the ship disappeared and was presumed to have sailed off. These events were reported to the master, Captain Lord, who was resting in his cabin. When the morning watch came on it was decided not to rouse the wireless operator. They then learnt that the *Titanic* had foundered and at 6 am steamed towards the scene of the disaster, arriving in the vicinity of the *Carpathia* at 8.30 am.

The immediate aftermath

The *Carpathia* sailed to New York and her arrival was the occasion of much public excitement and press speculation on both sides of the Atlantic (Fig. 3.4). The US Senate almost immediately set up its own committee of inquiry under the chairmanship of Senator William Alden Smith. The *Titanic* was an American-owned ship, the White Star Company having been

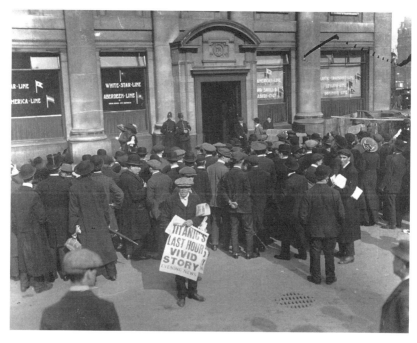

3.4 Londoners outside Oceanic House in Cockspur Street near Trafalgar Square read about the tragedy.

bought by J P Morgan before she was built. Morgan was due to travel on the maiden voyage but at the last moment cancelled his trip and went ashore, thereby making his own contribution to *Titanic* mythology.

Senator Smith's knowledge of ships and seafaring matters was exceedingly small, but this did not prevent him coming to positive conclusions about the cause of the tragedy: it was due primarily to overconfidence and indifference to danger on the part of Captain Smith, whilst Captain Lord of the *Californian* bore a heavy responsibility. All aspects of the disaster were criticised and only Captain Rostron of the *Carpathia* received any praise. The Senator did not improve Anglo–American relations.

The British formal investigation was led by a lawyer, Lord Mersea. It exonerated Captain Smith on the grounds that he was following normal practice, but said that had Captain Lord acted properly, many more lives could have been saved. Controversy over both these conclusions continues to the present day.

The officers and crew of the *Carpathia* were much praised for their rescue effort and several of their number received medals or decorations. The *Olympic* went into dock shortly afterwards, emerging with the double bottom extending up the sides of the hull and with rows of shining lifeboats along its decks. The Board of Trade regulations were amended, and lifeboat drill became a regular feature of the transatlantic (and other) crossings.

Finding the wreck

The development of techniques for underwater exploration began in earnest in the 1930s. One of the pioneers was Dr Piccard, who used a spherical diving shell known as the Bathyscape. This was the start of a long tradition of French underwater work. The US navy began to take a serious interest after the loss of the submarines *Theseus* in 1963 and *Scorpion* in 1968. The needs of the offshore oil and gas industry for exploration, inspection and maintenance gave further impetus to this development, leading to the current generation of submarines, which are mainly unmanned vehicles controlled from surface ships. Garzke *et al.*[2] gave an excellent review of developments up to 1992, starting with Alexander the Great, who is said to have descended into the waters of the Aegean sea in a glass bell in order to view the wonders of undersea life.

It is appropriate that the wreck of the *Titanic* was eventually located by a collaborative effort by French and US explorers. The French team first narrowed the field of search using a sonar scan, then Dr Ballard and his colleagues from Woods Hole Oceanographic Institution employed a remotely controlled camera sled *Argo* to examine the remaining area visually,[3] and in September 1985 finally located the wreck at a depth of 12 000 ft.

It came as a surprise that the remains of the ship were in two large pieces, 1970 ft apart. It had been generally supposed (although some eyewitnesses had said otherwise) that after colliding with the iceberg the ship sank substantially intact. This, indeed, was the conclusion of the Board of Inquiry. The distance between the two parts is about one-sixth of the water depth, suggesting that the separation took place some way below the surface. The bow portion is more or less intact, but the stern has been crushed into a tangled mass of wreckage.

Garzke et al.[2] suggest the following sequence of events:

1   Just before the final plunge, the stern was raised clear of the water at an angle of 45–60 degrees. This induced high stresses in the deck plating and girders, which were enhanced by the presence of the two heavy reciprocating engines.
2   The initial break probably started in 'B' deck between the compass platform and the third funnel. About this time the boilers in No 1 Boiler Room came loose and were forced up against the deck girders, allowing the sides to compress inwards.
3   The ship sank when only partially severed, but at some distance below the surface a final separation took place.
4   The forward portion was already flooded and pressures were equalised, so it did not suffer any significant damage due to water pressure. The stern portion on the other hand still contained air and was crushed as it descended.

This proposed sequence makes sense and conforms with the majority of eyewitness accounts.

The cause of the tragedy

The first question to answer is: how is it possible that four alert men were unable to see a major obstacle until it was too late to avoid it? They were experienced seamen, accustomed to the job of spotting ice, so it has to be concluded that the iceberg was not visible except at relatively close quarters. One of the lookouts in the crow's nest, Fleet, described it as a 'dark shadow on the water', and the other man, Lee, told the Mersea inquiry 'It was a dark mass that came through the haze and there was no white appearing until it was just close alongside the ship, and that was just a fringe at the top'.

Sir Ernest Shackleton, the polar explorer, explained this phenomenon to the inquiry. Exceptionally, an iceberg may melt or disintegrate in such a way that it becomes top heavy and capsizes. The underside, which is then exposed, appears black owing to contamination with earthy matter and porosity. He had twice seen such icebergs in the North Atlantic.

The other factor making for invisibility was the dead calm: there was not even a swell. Consequently, there was no ring of breakers around the berg. Lightoller suggested that it might be another 100 years before these two conditions occurred together again. He was almost certainly right because there had not been any sinking due to an iceberg on the transatlantic shipping lanes up to that time and there has not been another to this day. One ship, the *Hans Hedtoft* struck an iceberg in 1959 off the coast of Greenland and went down with the loss of all 95 passengers and crew. So although sinking through collision with an iceberg is a rare event, it could still happen even with the navigational aids available in the late 1950s.

As to whether the speed was too high: well, with hindsight, it was indeed so. But by prior standards it was quite normal to proceed at full speed through the ice, provided that visibility was good. Experience had indicated that this practice was safe provided that experienced lookouts were posted. Lord Mersea's assessment of the situation would seem to be a reasonable one.

As to the *Californian*: there is a fair body of opinion nowadays that would reject the charge that the Captain and crew were wilfully negligent. After all, they did steam at full speed through the ice to the disaster area on the following morning. And it did take over two hours to get there. So the notion that she could have averted the tragedy is open to question.

In fact it would seem, if the above analysis is correct, that the *Titanic* suffered the classic type of catastrophe where several unfavourable circumstances or events, each one of which has a low probability, coincide. The possibility that the ship would founder on its first voyage would have appeared to the passengers who set off from Southampton to be a virtual impossibility; and for good reason, for that is exactly what it was.

The brittle fracture theory

Following the discovery of the wreck, samples of the steel plate used in construction have been obtained and tested. The results showed that the notch-ductility of the material at 31 °F (the water temperature at the time of the sinking) was low; in other words the steel was notch-brittle. This fact led Garzke et al.[2] to suggest that brittle behaviour of the plate could have 'contributed to the hypothesised rivet or plate failures'. This rather modest suggestion has been much improved in press reports, for example in *The Times* of 17 September 1993:

> Maritime experts who presented their findings yesterday to the Society of Naval Architects and Marine Engineers in New York, blamed the rapid flooding on extensive cracks in the steel plates. . . . The team attributed the cracking to 'brittle fracture' in which low-grade steel breaks violently when cold, rather than bending . . . better quality steel might have kept her afloat for another two hours.[4]

In fact, there is not the slightest evidence that brittle cracking had anything to do with the *Titanic* disaster. When steel is in a notch-brittle condition, a plate containing a crack and subject to a tensile stress may fail suddenly at a relatively low value of stress. However, if an uncracked specimen of the same steel is subject to a normal tensile test at the same temperature it will fail in a normal ductile manner, although it will stretch plastically somewhat less than a more notch-ductile steel. Likewise, when subject to a bending load, it will, in the absence of a notch or crack, bend and not break. It is only when there is a notch or crack of sufficient length already present in the material that it will behave in a brittle way.

The wreck itself provided clear evidence of ductile behaviour. The stern portion was severely damaged by implosion, but did not break up. The forward portion, apart from local areas, is bent but not broken. And according to most witnesses, the ship went down in one piece, suggesting that the bottom plates must have bent initially, and then parted after she was below the surface.

The difficulty, indeed, is to explain why she remained afloat so long after such a severe impact. The Harland and Wolff designer, Edward Wilding, calculated that the area of leakage was 144 square inches. The length of the damage, as noted previously, was reckoned to be about 250 ft. If the gap had been uniform along this distance it would have been about 3/64 inch or 1.2 mm wide. Suppose that there were six gaps each 2 ft in length, then the average width would be 1 in. These figures are consistent with a model in which the plating was buckled sufficiently to break the rivets and displace the caulking. In such a case the rivets would have failed or would have been torn out regardless of their ductility. The real problem seems to have been the length of the damaging contact, which meant that five or six of the forward compartments were flooded.

The report in the London *Times* newspaper implied that a better grade of steel could have been used to build the ship, and this could have saved lives by keeping the ship afloat for another two hours. In fact, there was at the time only one grade of shipbuilding steel. The required properties of this grade were specified by Lloyd's Register of Shipping, which also inspected and approved the steelworks and witnessed the testing of samples from each melt. The suggestion that inferior material was used is entirely without foundation.

Riveted ships do not suffer from catastrophic brittle failure. The brittle fracture problem arose some 30 years after the building of the *Titanic*, when the first all-welded ships went into use. With a monolithic hull, a running crack could split the ship in two; in a riveted ship the crack only got as far as the edge of the plate in which it initiated. Such localised cracking did occur from time to time, but would always require an initiating defect, usually a fatigue crack. Fatigue cracks take some time to develop. The *Titanic* was a new ship, so even localised brittle fractures would have been highly improbable. It may be concluded that although the hull plates of the *Titanic* were in a notch-brittle condition at the time of her encounter with the iceberg, they were very unlikely to have failed in a brittle fashion; all the evidence suggests that they bent and did not break.

Ferry disasters: introduction

Ferry accidents can be particularly distressing because the victims are often ordinary people going on holiday, visiting friends or relatives or simply enjoying a cruise without any thought of dire consequences. The loss of over 800 lives including those of pensioners and children when the *Estonia* capsized and sank in the Baltic Sea in September 1994 was particularly tragic.

So far as loss of life is concerned, the world's worst shipping accident occurred when the Philippine ferry boat *Dona Paz* was in collision with an oil tanker. In the ensuing fire nearly 4400 people were killed. However, safety on ferry boats in the Philippines is very far from that in the developed countries. The average annual death toll for the period 1980–89 was 620. In Britain, a country with a similar population, the average death rate of passengers in ferry operations from 1950 to 1988 was 7 per year.[5] Evidently the level of risk in these two areas is very different and they need to be treated separately. The comparison will have a special interest. As noted elsewhere, the statistics quoted in this book relate primarily to industrialised countries. The Philippine ferries (of which J Spouge has provided an excellent account[6]) are an interesting example of such operations in a developing country. A similar disparity applies in the case of death rates due to road accidents, as noted in Chapter 1. In Ethiopia, for example, the death rate from this cause was, in the 1990s, over a hundred times that in Great Britain.

Ferry disasters: the Estonia

At 7 pm on Tuesday, 27 September 1994 the motorship *Estonia* left the port of Tallinn in Estonia bound for Stockholm. The *Estonia* was a roll-on, roll-off (ro-ro) ferry which had a capacity of 460 cars and space for 2000 passengers. She was equipped with both bow and stern doors, the bow door being of the visor type: that is to say it hinged upwards to open. The vessel itself had been built in Papenburg, Germany, in 1980.

At about 1.20 am on the morning of 28 September the third engineer Margus Treu, who was in the engine room at the time, heard two or three strong blows that shook the whole ship. Shortly afterwards the vessel heeled suddenly, throwing passengers off their feet. For a time the list stabilised, such that some of the passengers had time to dress and to climb up on deck. Then, about 15 minutes later, the ship turned on its side and sank.

There was no time for an orderly evacuation and in any event power was lost when the ship first heeled, so lifeboats could not have been lowered. A number of liferafts were flung into the sea and these were the means by which some of the passengers survived. The weather was squally with waves up to 30 ft. In several cases individuals were washed off their raft and had to fight their way back. The first survivors were picked up by the ferry boats *Mariella* and *Symphony*, which were nearby. Then at first light helicopters took off from the mainland to help in the rescue operation. Altogether 140 were saved, most being young men, but 852 lives were lost, making this the worst peacetime ferry disaster in European waters.

The vessel lay at a depth of 230 ft near the island of Uto, off the coast of Finland. As soon as the sea became calmer, video cameras mounted on underwater craft were sent down. In addition to the outer door, ferries are required by the classification societies to have an inner door, which is held in place by hydraulic clamps and which forms the main barrier against the ingress of water. The video pictures were clear and showed that the outer door of the *Estonia* had been torn off and was missing, whilst the inner door had been forced open such that there was a gap of about 3 ft along its upper edge. A later search revealed the missing door on the sea-bed at a distance of about one mile from the main part of the wreck.

Subsequently, an international commission of inquiry was set up, with representation from the three countries directly concerned: Estonia, Finland and Sweden. Tests were carried out and it was determined that in heavy seas, the outer door would have been subject to exceptionally high loads acting in an upward direction. The bolting system that had been provided was inadequate to withstand these forces and in the opinion of the commission these bolts should have been six times stronger. It was found that other Baltic ferries had suffered failures of visor door fasteners, but in these cases the ship had found shelter before any disastrous failure occurred. The crew of the *Estonia* were also criticised for proceeding at full speed in severe weather: other ferries had reduced speed in order to avoid excessive loading on the doors.

The shipbuilder rejected the commission's findings about the strength of the fasteners and claimed that the hull was breached in some other way. He thought that the failure could have been due to poor maintenance. Poor maintenance may indeed have contributed to the disaster, but there is little doubt that failure of the visor was the primary cause.

The safety of roll-on, roll-off ferries

The loss of the *Estonia* confirmed the worst predictions of those who believed that this type of ship was, because of the design, unstable and liable to capsize rapidly and catastrophically if water invaded the main vehicle deck. This loss occurred not very long after the International Maritime Organisation (an agency of the United Nations) had agreed that following a collision, ferries should be capable of remaining afloat and upright for at least 45 minutes, leaving sufficient time (in theory, at least) for the passengers to escape. The agreement failed to obtain full international support, nor, as will be seen later, would it be realistic to expect this to be so. Nevertheless, some countries have adopted it as an objective. The *Estonia* disaster has shown that there is much work to be done before this objective is achieved.

Roll-on, roll-off ferries were developed during the post-1945 period from the vessels that were used for the Normandy and other seaborne invasions by Allied forces. Indeed some of the early ferries used adapted LSTs (landing ship, tank). They are characterised by shallow draught (necessary to serve ferry ports), a vehicle deck which runs the length of the ship and is normally open, and access doors with a low freeboard to give a level or gently sloped loading ramp. Early versions had side doors, but these cause difficulties in loading and unloading, so that most of the contemporary designs have bow and stern doors. There are two types of door, the visor and the clam types. The visor, as tragically demonstrated in the case of the *Estonia*, is less safe because wave motion tends to open it. The clam type is flat-faced and closes by hinging upwards. It is more difficult to make watertight and is less elegant, but is less subject to weather damage. Neither type is expected to be completely watertight and the water seal is provided by an inner door, as noted earlier.

In the larger boats it is possible for vehicles to turn through 180° and the bow door can be eliminated. This greatly reduces the risk, but at the expense of speed in turn-round. For the future it is likely that vessels operating in rough seas such as the Baltic and North Sea will have a stern door only. New vessels for North Sea operations have been so constructed.

Ro-ro ferry ships may become unstable for a number of reasons, including shallow draught, low freeboard and the long vehicle deck.

Flooding of the vehicle deck is the most-feared event, because it can result in a very rapid capsize, such that no proper evacuation is possible. When a substantial volume of water enters the car deck it flows either to one side or the other, causing a rapid heel. After the initial movement the vessel will stabilise temporarily, but will then continue to heel and finally capsize or, in shallow water, settle on its side.

This type of flooding is a special feature of ro-ro ferries but is only one of the many accidents to which these vessels may be subject, as will be seen below.

The record of ro-ro accidents

Since the Second World War, ferries in industrial countries have experienced seven major incidents resulting in the sinking of a ro-ro vessel. These are listed, together with a brief summary of the causes, sequence of events and casualty rate, in Table 3.1. Two of the seven were due to flooding through the bow door. One of these, the *Herald of Free Enterprise* (Fig. 3.5), was a loss caused by gross maloperation and the procedures of the operating company concerned have been modified so that a repetition of such an accident with its ships is highly improbable. Such procedures do not, however, offer any protection against the *Estonia* type of accident and it remains to be determined how this problem may be resolved. Of the other sinkings, one was due to failure of the stern door and one to side doors being stove in; in other words the bow door is not the only vulnerable point. One sinking was due to a collision, but apart from that of the *Herald of Free Enterprise* the remainder were all primarily caused by severe weather or heavy seas. In all cases the ships finally capsized and sank, but except for the *Estonia* and the *Herald of Free Enterprise*, where there was a massive inundation of the vehicle deck, they all remained afloat long enough to organise an evacuation and, in some cases, to launch the lifeboats. Thus, most ferry sinkings (about 70%) were due to normal shipping-type hazards. On the other hand, 85% (1103 of 1295) of the deaths, as presently recorded, were due to flooding of the vehicle deck. For European ferries this remains the most important problem.

Philippines ferries: the Dona Paz *disaster*

The Republic of the Philippines is a country consisting of an archipelago of 7000 islands, of which 880 or so are inhabited. Most of the population lives on the eight largest islands. Following independence in 1946 there was a succession of presidents but after the election of President Marcos in 1965 a period of rapid economic development occurred. Insurgency in the

Table 3.1 Major European ferry sinkings (in part from Spouge[5])

Date	Ship	Location	Cause of flooding	Where flooded	Sequence of events	Number on board	Dead
1953	*Princess Victoria*	Irish Sea	Large wave burst open stern door in rough seas	Car deck and starboard engine room	Listed, reaching 45° in 4h. Capsized and sank after 5h. Ship abandoned	172	134
1966	*Skagerak*	Skagerak	Heavy seas stove in side doors	Engine room	Sudden heel, cargo shifted. Ship abandoned except for 11 crew. Capsized and sank when under tow	144	1
1968	*Wahine*	Wellington, New Zealand	Grounded on rocks in severe weather	Bow and stern below decks	Remained afloat for 5½h, then started to heel. Capsized and sank after 7½h. Abandoned	735	51
1980	*Zenobia*	Cyprus	Failure of autopilot, causing list	General	Passengers and crew evacuated. Vessel capsized and sank during attempted salvage	151	0
1982	*European Gateway*	Off Felixstowe, UK	Rammed by ro-ro ferry *Speedlink Vanguard*	Engine room	Heeled to 40° in 3 min at which point bilge grounded and she rolled on her side in 10–20 min	70	6
1987	*Herald of Free Enterprise*	Zeebrugge	Bow doors not closed prior to sailing	Vehicle deck	Bow wave high enough to flood lower vehicle deck. Heeled to 30°, then paused for few seconds, finally grounding on her side	539	193
1994	*Estonia*	Off coast of Finland	Outer bow door torn off in heavy seas, inner door forced open	Vehicle deck	Vessel heeled suddenly, stabilised for few minutes, capsized and sank in 15–20 min	about 1050	852

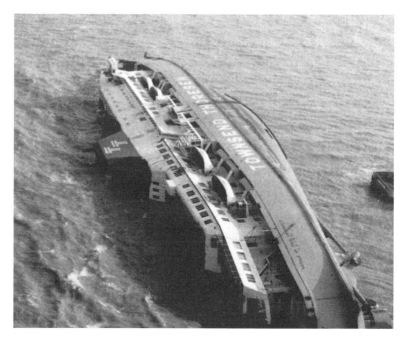

3.5 The *Herald of Free Enterprise* capsized outside Zeebrugge harbour.

north and Muslim separatism in the south led to increasingly despotic rule by Marcos and the economy stagnated. After the fall of Marcos and the restoration of democracy there was some recovery. However, the country remains very poor, with a (theoretical) daily minimum wage (in 1990) of 114 pesos, equivalent to about US$5.50. The main economic activity centres around agriculture, forestry and fishing, and more recently the mining of metallic ores. The population is about 60 million and, because of the lack of industrial development, many seek work abroad, as seamen, hotel staff and servants.

Poverty also means that travel between the islands is almost entirely by ferry; only a small number of people can afford to go by air. Ferry boats are of all sizes. The smaller islands, where port facilities are lacking, are served by outrigger canoes capable of carrying up to 50 people, and by other smaller craft. The rest of the fleet consists mainly of second-hand vessels (such as that shown in Fig. 3.6), often purchased in Japan, with an average age of about 20 years. There are a number of ro-ro vessels, but outside the main cities there are few cars and the vehicle decks are often used for cargo and passengers.

The *Dona Paz* was a three-deck passenger ferry boat of 2324 registered tonnage and with an authorised passenger capacity of 1518. It was built in

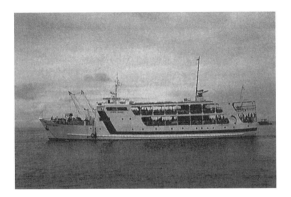

3.6 *Sweet Heart,* built 1965, registered tonnage 475, capacity 400 passengers.

Japan in 1963 and went into service in the Philippines in 1975, at which time it lost classification. In 1979 it was gutted by fire but was reconstructed and returned to service. On 20 December 1987 it was crossing from Tacloban to Manila, loaded with over 4000 passengers returning for the Christmas holiday. During the night it collided with the tanker *Vector.* Both vessels were engulfed in fire and sank, with the loss of (it is estimated) 4376 lives.

The tanker carried 1130 tonnes of gasoline, kerosene and diesel fuels. It was operating without a licence, without a lookout and without a properly qualified master. Two of the 13 crew managed to escape and were picked up by another ferry. On the *Dona Paz* most of the passengers were trapped in the burning ship; only 24 were able to get away and were rescued by the same ferry. The *Dona Paz* had no radio, and it was 16 hours before a rescue operation was mounted. By this time it was far too late.

The accident records

Statistics for fatalities on Philippines ferries are derived mainly from newspaper reports. Table 3.2 lists the information available for the period 1980–89. The number of fatalities listed in this table totals 6224 so that the annual loss is over 600 persons. Spouge[6] estimates 17 million crossings per year for Philippines ferries in the late 1980s, so that the fatality rate at that time was 36.6 deaths per million departures, over one hundred times that for British ferries.

Comparisons

Such disasters and the generally high risk of ferry travel are accepted in the Philippines because of the generally high accident rate amongst the

Table 3.2 Ferry accidents in the Philippines, 1980–89[6]

Date	Ship	Tonnage	Cause of loss	Number on board	Dead
April 1980	*Don Juan*	2300	Collision, sank	Over 1000	Over 121
July 1981	*Juan*	1530	Fire	Over 458	Over 57
Sept 1981	*Sweet Trip* (ro-ro)	500	Sank	Not known	1
June 1982	*Queen Helen*	500	Sabotage, explosion, fire	484	48
March 1983	*Sweet Name* (ro-ro)	580	Collision, explosion, fire	400	27
May 1983	*Dona Florentina*	2100	Fire, beached	884	0
Nov 1983	*Dona Cassandra*	487	Capsized in storm	396	177
Nov 1983	*Santo Nino*	Not Known	Capsized	Not Known	12
Jan 1984	*Nashra*	Not Known	Steering gear failure, capsized	Not Known	52
Jan 1984	*Asia Singapore*	720	Capsized in port during storm	568	21
Oct 1984	*Venus*	746	Sank in storm	351	137
Dec 1985	*Asuncion*	141	Sank	About 200	136
April 1986	*Dona Josephina* (ro-ro)	1000	Flooded, sank	414	194
Sept 1987	*Kolambugan*	770	Fire, sank	150	0
Dec 1987	*Dona Paz*	2324	Collision, fire, sank	4400	4376
April 1988	*Balangiga*	Not Known	Sank in typhoon	148	63
Oct 1988	*Dona Marilyn*	2855	Sank in typhoon	481	284
Dec 1988	*Rosalia*	Not Known	Sank in storm	410	400
Dec 1988	*RCJ*	Not Known	Sank in storm	53	51
Jan 1989	*Jem III*	Not Known	Capsized	Over 190	Over 60
Nov 1989	*Jalmaida*	Not Known	Sank in storm	Over 180	Over 7

population. Large numbers of outriggers, pump boats and motor launches that also operate as ferries suffer accidents and it has been estimated that the total loss of life at sea in the Philippines is between 20 000 and 40 000 per year.[7] By comparison, the losses on the large boats are small. Part of the problem is that the area is affected by typhoons, but in the main it is due to unseaworthy boats with unreliable engines carrying too many passengers.[6]

Such conditions and fatality rates apply to other poor countries. A process upset in a chemical plant located at Bhopal, India, resulted in the emission of poisonous gases. The number of deaths resulting from the accident was 3031. The reason for the excessive loss of life was that people were camping around the perimeter of the plant hoping for work or some other benefit. Life is cheap in such countries; literally so, because the Indian government offered the equivalent of about US$800 compensation for each life lost at Bhopal, whilst the owners of the *Dona Paz* paid just over US$900 to relatives of those who died in that disaster. These figures may be compared with the 1974 Athens Convention compensation limit of about US$60 000 per passenger, which itself is low by current standards.

From every point of view, therefore, it is necessary to treat statistics for accidents in third world countries quite separately from those for Europe and North America. The most important problem for European ferries is a technical one; how to improve the safety of roll-on, roll-off vessels. This problem is wholly irrelevant in the Philippines. Moreover, if all the figures are lumped together, ro-ro sinkings account for only a small proportion of fatalities; treated separately, the opposite is the case. Figure 3.7, which is a frequency–consequence plot comparing British and Philippines ferry losses, underlines the need for separate treatment.

It was noted in Chapter 1 that the fatality rate in road accidents was much higher in undeveloped countries than in Europe, Japan and the USA, and that in some cases the ratio between the two rates could be 100 or more.

It appears that a similar state of affairs applies, although to a lesser degree, in the case of air transport. Harris,[8] quoting from an article in the *Guardian* newspaper, gives figures for the rate of loss of aircraft, expressed in numbers per million departures. These indicate a significantly higher loss rate in the less-developed countries. However, in this field the overwhelming majority of flights take place from and within developed countries, so worldwide figures are unlikely to be affected to any significant extent by such differences.

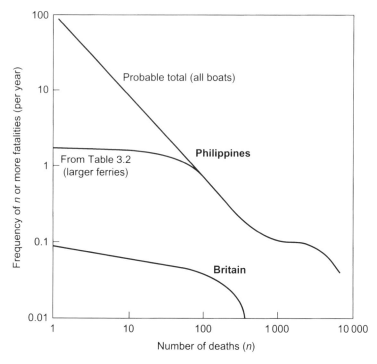

3.7 Frequency–consequence curve for ferry casualties, comparing those in the Philippines with those sailing from British ports.

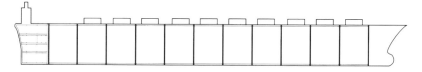

3.8 Diagrammatic cross-section of a bulk carrier (after Anon[11]).

Bulk carriers: the Derbyshire and others

Bulk carriers are vessels designed to carry very large quantities of cargo such as grain, coal or iron ore. In effect, they are rectangular boxes divided into compartments, with machinery and crew accommodation tacked on the stern, as shown diagrammatically in Fig. 3.8. Typically such vessels could be 1000 ft long, 100 ft high and 150 ft wide, and contain 30 000 tons of welded steelwork. Bulkheads are usually corrugated in form and there is a complex system of internal stiffeners, attached to the steel plates by fillet welds. In many cases the material used has been Lloyd's Grade A steel or equivalent. This is a general-purpose grade and is not subject to impact testing.

The rate at which these large vessels are lost is a matter of great concern. Between 1973 and 1996 the losses amounted to 375. The fatality rate is likewise disturbing; for the same period it was about 150 per year, one-fifth of the total average loss rate for all shipping. Furthermore, little is known about the manner in which these ships foundered and whether or not there is a common design fault. Technical aspects of this problem are reviewed by Jubb,[9] and Faith[10] describes three of the losses in detail.

To date the most thorough investigation of a casualty is that of the *Derbyshire*. This 170 000 ton ship had been built in 1976 at the Swan Hunter shipyard on the River Tyne. In September 1980 she sank during a tropical storm in the South China sea whilst *en route* from Seattle to Yokohama with a cargo of iron ore. All 44 persons on board were lost. No radio distress call was received, so it is assumed that a sudden catastrophic event occurred. Relatives of the deceased believed at the time that there had been a structural failure due to a design fault, such that the aft portion of the ship had parted from the forward cargo-carrying part. Some engineers shared this view, noting that, amongst other evidence, brittle cracks had been found in the deck plating of one of the *Derbyshire*'s sister ships. Accordingly the families' association, with financial support from the International Transport Federation, set up an underwater search. In June 1994 the wreck was located at a depth of 14 000 ft (just over two and a half miles), scattered over a distance of a mile from east to west. At this point the available funds ran out. The British government then financed a further search by the Woods Hole Oceanographic Institute of Massachusetts. The wreck was fully mapped and it was found that the stern portion was separated from the forward part by a distance of 600 m. This was a clear indication that the ship had sunk in one piece. If the stern portion had separated at the surface it is most unlikely that the forward part, which contained numbers of watertight bulkheads, would have sunk at the same time. It would have remained afloat for some time, driven by the wind, and the two wrecks would have been widely separated. Thus, the structural weakness hypothesis was discounted and attention concentrated instead on the potential weakness of the hatch covers. The strength of these items was calculated to be about one-tenth that of the deck itself. One small hatch cover was missing and others were stove-in (although this could have happened as the ship was sinking). The sudden inundation of water into a cargo hold might well cause the ship to dive like a submarine, precluding any distress signal.

In 1975 there was an incident on Lake Superior in North America that had some features in common with the loss of the *Derbyshire*. The bulk carrier *Edmund Fitzgerald* was caught in a severe storm and lost her radar, so that it was not possible to fix the ship's position. Accordingly, the captain requested assistance from a sister ship, the *Arthur Anderson*. Later, the captain of the *Fitzgerald* reported that the ship was taking in water and was listing. Then came a message to the effect that they were 'holding on'. Shortly after this there was a snow flurry that blocked the radar on the *Anderson*, and when this cleared there was no sign of the *Fitzgerald*. There was no 'Mayday' signal: the ship sank suddenly with the loss of all twenty-nine crew.

The US Coastguard set up an investigation team, which examined the wreck using underwater equipment. The *Fitzgerald* had gone down in 500 ft of water and access was good. The forward portion of the ship was the right way up, but the stern was detached and keel uppermost. It was concluded that the vessel had not capsized and that it had started to sink in one piece, the breakup having occurred during the descent. But most significantly, number 5 hatch cover was missing. The other hatch covers were in place, but some of the fastening clamps were damaged. It was concluded that the ship had taken in water through hatch covers where the clamps were not fully effective, and then, being low in the water, waves breaking over the deck had torn off number 5 hatch cover. The ship then foundered suddenly, as in the case of the *Derbyshire*.

It should not be thought that hatch covers are the only source of weakness in bulk carriers. As one of the team investigating the loss of the *Edmund Fitzgerald* pointed out, hatch covers do not normally cause problems.

There is also the case of the *Flare*.[10] This was a 400-ft bulk carrier that in January 1998 was proceeding empty from Rotterdam to Montreal to pick up a cargo of grain. She was travelling in light ballast, such that the deck was some 60 ft above sea level. The sea off the coast of Newfoundland was rough and the crew became concerned because cracks appeared in the hull. At 4.37 am on the morning of 16 January 1998, after sailing through heavy seas, the ship broke in two. All the crew were in the after section and most were asleep. By the time that they got up on deck the stern portion was listing and sinking. One lifeboat was washed overboard, whilst the other was high in the air. When this was released it fell into the sea and capsized. Six men jumped into the icy water, swam to the upturned lifeboat and climbed aboard. Two were washed off but the remaining four were rescued. Twenty-one crew members were drowned.

The cargo section of the ship remained afloat for two days after the breakup. There is little doubt that this failure resulted from fatigue cracking, resulting from the unusual configuration of a light bow section and a heavy stern, exposed to cyclic loading in rough seas. In such a case it is of no consequence whether the eventual fracture was brittle or ductile in character because it would have happened regardless.

These case histories point to two possible modes by which bulk carriers could suffer a catastrophic failure: loss of a hatch cover and severe fatigue loading. It must not be assumed, however, that these are the only types of failure. The case of the roll-on roll-off ferries must be borne in mind; whilst the most obvious and most catastrophic type of failure is that of the access doors, there are a number of other causes of loss, as will be evident from Table 3.1.

Catastrophes in the oil and gas production industry

The Alexander L Kielland accident

The floating objects that have been used for offshore oil and gas production started as modified barges or ships, but have progressively departed from the norm and some of the more recent developments look very unlike a conventional ship. The *Alexander L Kielland* was a semi-submersible drilling platform that had been adapted for use as an accommodation platform serving various individual production units in the Norwegian section of the North Sea.

Semi-submersible drilling rigs originated in the USA during the early 1960s. The object of this development was to provide more stable conditions than could be obtained in a drill ship, such that operations could be continued under more severe weather conditions. They consist of two or more submerged pontoons supporting a structure on which is mounted the operating platform and drilling equipment. It will be self-evident that a rig that obtains its buoyancy from submerged pontoons will be much less subject to wave motion than a surface ship. The first semi-submersible was *Blue Water I* which was delivered in 1962, followed by *Ocean Driller* in 1963 and *Ocean Queen* in 1965. Initially, these developments proceeded empirically. However, in 1978 the American Bureau of Shipping published a set of rules for the construction of mobile offshore units, followed by Det Norske Veritas and Lloyd's Register of Shipping, which published general guidelines in 1970 and 1972 respectively. Prior to the *Alexander L Kielland* disaster the record for semi-submersibles had been good. Two had been lost; *Transocean 3*, which capsized and sank after a structural failure in 1974, and *Seaco 135-C*, which was destroyed by fire following a blowout in January 1980.

The Pentagone rigs

In 1963 the Institut Français du Pétrole signed a cooperative agreement with Neptune, an oil exploration subsidiary of the Schlumberger group, to develop a design for a five-pontoon semi-submersible drilling rig. This led to the construction of the first Pentagone rig, P 81, which was delivered to Neptune in June 1969. In 1970 this company, together with various other organisations, reviewed the original design and came up with a number of modifications. These developments were incorporated in a new rig, P 82, which was constructed in Brownsville, Texas. This formed the basis for a further nine Pentagones, six of which were constructed in France and three in Finland. The *Alexander L Kielland* was the seventh of this group, numbered P 89, and was delivered in July 1976. The general layout of these rigs is shown (complete with derrick) in Fig. 3.9. Figure 3.10 is a sketch of the deck in plan view in relation to the location of the columns. This diagram also indicates the location of lifeboats and other rescue equipment. The various structural members were dimensioned to withstand the static loading associated with a maximum wave height of 30 m. There was no attempt to design against fatigue loading. At the Commission of Enquiry hearings, the designers claimed that this mode of fracture had been taken into account in the design of the structural details and the selection of geometric form and quality of materials.

It was necessary to tow the rig from one location to the other by tugs, the bow of the vessel being column C and the stern lying between columns A and E. Once in position it was fixed by ten anchors, two being attached to each column by wire hawsers having a diameter of 2.75 in and a breaking load of 310 tonnes. The position could be altered by operating winches mounted on the top of the columns. Screw propellers were fitted to each column and by operating these it was possible to modify the tension in the anchor lines.

The rig was originally developed with accommodation and rescue equipment for 80 persons. These facilities were expanded stepwise over a period of time by the addition of extra modules so that by March/April 1978 there were sleeping quarters for 318 men, with a mess hall (made by building several modules together) and two cinemas. The rescue equipment consisted of 7 lifeboats, 16 rafts under davits (launchable rafts) and 12 throw-overboard rafts. The lifeboats could hold 50 persons and the liferafts held 20 persons each, giving a theoretical availability of 910. This was the position also at the time of the accident except that four of the launchable rafts were ashore for maintenance.

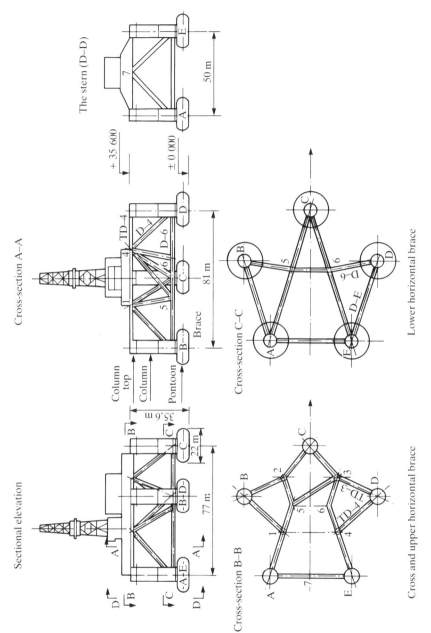

3.9 Plan and section of Pentagone-type semi-submersible rig.[11]

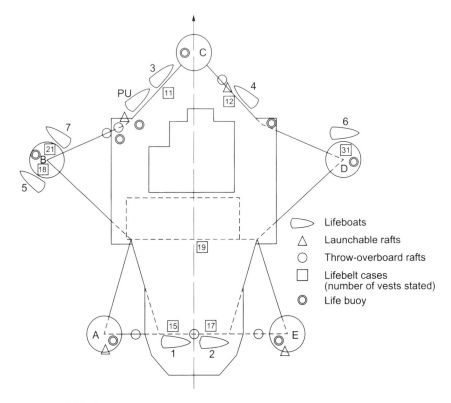

3.10 Diagrammatic plan view of *Alexander L Kielland* showing location of rescue equipment.[11]

The accident

For nine months prior to the accident *Alexander L Kielland* had been anchored close to the production platform *Edda 2/7 C*. Anchors were attached to all columns except column C, which was located nearest to the production platform. Contact between the two platforms was maintained by a movable walkway. In bad weather this walkway was hoisted on board the *Alexander L Kielland*, which was then winched away from the *Edda 2/7 C* by slacking the anchor wires on columns B and D and tightening those on A and E.

On Thursday, 27 March 1980 the weather was indeed poor. The wind speed was 36–45 mph and the wave height 20–26 ft. Accordingly, it was decided to move away from *Edda 2/7 C* by means of the winches. This was accomplished without incident by 5.50 pm. A few minutes before 6.30 pm those on board felt a sudden impact followed by trembling. At first this was thought to be due to a wave, but shortly afterwards there was a further impact and the platform shook and started to heel. The heeling continued until it reached an angle of 35°, at which point the radio operator sent out an emergency message 'Mayday, Mayday, *Kielland* is capsizing'. For a time the list stabilised, although the platform continued to take water through ventilators and other openings in the deck. One anchor wire, on B column, remained intact, but strained like a violin string. Eventually, at 6.53 pm, a little more than 20 minutes after the collapse started, the wire snapped and the platform overturned and floated upside down in the water.

Evacuation and rescue

Immediately before the accident most of the men were either in the mess hall or in the cinemas, and very few in the bedrooms, which were located aft. The heeling, which was due to the failure of the brace D6 and disintegration of column D, was a sudden collapse, which was arrested when part of the platform became submerged. As a result, most of those on board were thrown to one side of the room in which they had been sitting. From later medical evidence, however, it would seem that only a few were seriously injured at this time. Most were able to make their way on deck, although with some difficulty.

Twenty-six men escaped aft, where lifeboats No 1 and 2 were located below the helideck. Because of the list, No 2 boat was under water but No 1 was clear. Its engine was started and when no more people appeared, the boat was launched. The lifeboats were provided with a release wire. After it was afloat, pulling this wire was supposed to open the hooks that attached the boat to the davits. This failed to operate, and while one man was pulling frantically at the release wire, another attacked the forward hook with an axe. Then suddenly the forward hook released itself, but by this time they had been thrown back on to the platform, with some damage to the superstructure. The back of the wheelhouse was stove in, and whilst they were stranded one man was able to reach through the hole and release the other hook. The boat then floated clear of the wreck. It was seaworthy and the engine was operating, but radio communication was difficult. Eventually, at about 1.20 am the following morning, they were spotted by two of the supply ships. However, since the lifeboat was in good shape it was decided not to transfer the men to these ships and they were rescued by helicopter, the last man being winched up at 5.00 am in the morning. The weather continued to be bad, visibility was poor and throughout this protracted operation men were seasick and very cold.

Most of those who managed to escape from the mess room, cinemas and quarters made for the highest point, which was column B. Lifeboat No 5 was located here, but only 14 men got on board; others thought it would be crushed against the crossbrace as it was lowered. In the event it never was lowered, but was flung into the sea bottom up as the platform capsized. Fortunately the hooks were released and the boat drifted away from the upturned platform. Some of the survivors from the platform swam over to the lifeboat and by superhuman efforts, helped by those inside, managed to right it. A further 19 people were then able to board the craft. It was not possible to start the engine and the radio did not work, but at 7.30 pm in the evening the boat was found by the supply ship *Normand Skipper*. Twelve men were taken on board the ship by an entry net before the operation became too hazardous, and the ship stood off. The other men were rescued by helicopter between 2.30 am and 4.00 am in the morning.

Of the remaining lifeboats, No 2, which had been already submerged, went down with the platform and No 6 was lost when D column collapsed. No 3 was located on the port side and was lowered with seven or eight persons on board. The launch was successful but it was only possible to release the aft hook. The boat was pushed under the platform but was then lifted up by a big wave and landed on top of the winch on C column. Those on board managed to escape and, except for one man who was injured, were eventually rescued.

No 4 lifeboat was lowered but was crushed and there were no survivors. No 7 boat was launched but it capsized. A number of those aboard were able to get through the side hatches, and of these, three were rescued.

Altogether 59 survivors were picked up by helicopter from the lifeboats. The other 30 were rescued from liferafts, or swam to the operating platform, or were rescued by the supply ships.

The rescue helicopters and ships had serious difficulties owing to poor visibility and, to a minor extent, because of problems with the winches on the helicopters. Nevertheless, they picked up all those who were on rafts or lifeboats, whilst the ships and *Edda 2/7 C* rescued men from the sea. The number of rescue units increased during the operation, such that eventually the Norwegian authorities requested that an RAF Nimrod aircraft should co-ordinate air movements, whilst a Dutch warship controlled shipping. This arrangement seems to have worked very well.

Hydrophones

It has already been mentioned that the *Alexander L Kielland* was originally designed as a drilling platform. As such, it was equipped with hydrophones. These instruments pick up an acoustic signal from a source located in the well and enable the platform to be positioned accurately. It so happened that at the time of the accident, the platform was being prepared for drilling operations, so the hydrophones were by no means superfluous. These instruments were mounted on the lower horizontal braces and, in particular, there was one on brace D6 which, as shown in Fig. 3.9, joined column D with a node in the brace between columns C and E. The location of this hydrophone is illustrated in greater detail in Fig. 3.11(a). The hydrophone itself was mounted inside a cylindrical fitting which was attached to the brace (Fig. 3.11(b)). The cylinder was made by rolling plate to the required diameter and joining the edges with a butt weld. A matching hole was cut out of the brace and the cylinder fixed in position by one internal and one external fillet weld, each of 6 mm throat thickness. The hydrophone and its mounting were classified by the designer as an instrument and therefore no stress analysis was made of this detail.

The collapse started as the result of a fatigue failure of brace D6, and this in turn was initiated at the toe of the fillet welds. The crack started at the 12 and 6 o'clock positions, looking at the hydrophone fitting with the brace horizontal. It then propagated around the circumference of the brace until the remaining ligament was too small to sustain the applied stress, when it suffered a sudden catastrophic failure. It has been estimated that the parting of this ligament took place in less than one-hundredth of a second. As a result, the remaining braces connecting column D were subject to dynamic loading which had the effect of amplifying the loads to which they would have been subject under static conditions. These braces were not designed to operate safely in the absence of brace D6, so they failed, also in a very short time (see Chapter 4 for some proposals about the nature of this process). Inevitably column D then collapsed. The failures were partly shear failures, partly flat fractures, and in most cases occurred in two places, close to the nodes or to the junction with the column. There is no suggestion that inferior material contributed greatly to these later failures; on the contrary, later testing of the material showed that it met specification requirements except for a few trivial deviations and was generally of good notch-ductility at the temperature then prevailing (between 4 and 6 °C).

The appearance of the fracture in the brace D6 is shown in Fig. 3.12. There were two independent initiation sites, No I from the outside fillet weld and No II from the inside fillet. Such points of initiation of fatigue cracking are typical of a fillet-welded attachment exposed to an alternating tensile stress. Fillet welds reduce the fatigue strength of steels in two ways. First, the profile of the weld causes a stress concentration. Secondly, a crack or slag-filled intrusion, commonly up to 0.5 mm in depth, is usually to be found near the toe of the fillet. This defect is responsible for the major part of the reduction in fatigue life and it is current practice to grind the toe of fillet welds in critical areas to remove such defects.

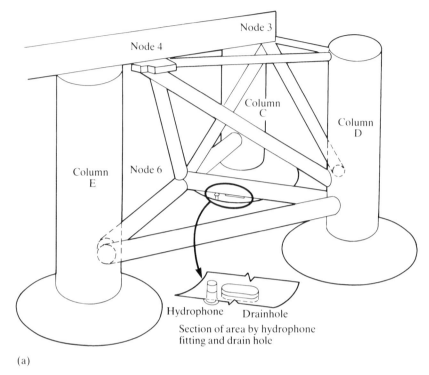

(a)

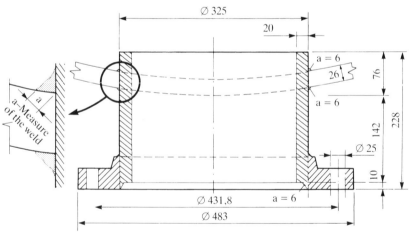

(b)

3.11 The hydrophone fitting on brace D6 of the *Alexander L Kielland*: (a) location of fitting; (b) sectional elevation with nominal dimensions in mm. The dimension A is the throat thickness of the attachment weld, specified to be 6 mm.

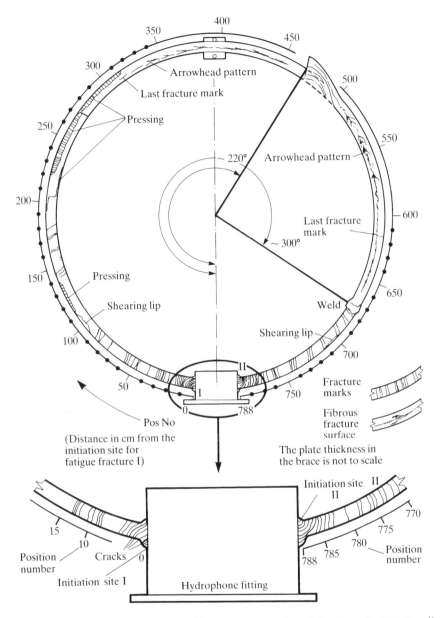

3.12 Surface appearance of fracture in brace D6 of the *Alexander L Kielland*.[11]

Fatigue fracture appearance

The general appearance of the first part of the crack, as shown in the sketch, is characteristic of a fatigue failure. There is little or no reduction in thickness and the surface is marked periodically with striations. These represent either a slight change in direction or a change in the crack growth rate. Examination under the microscope shows additional features; in particular, there are fine striations which are generally assumed to indicate individual load cycles.

After the first 300 mm or so on either side of the hydrophone fitting the fracture appearance changes, indicating that it was growing in leaps, giving a coarse and fibrous fracture surface. Finally, the last third of the circumference has a woody appearance with chevron (herringbone) marks which are typical of fast, unstable crack propagation. These various modes of failure are discussed more fully in Chapter 4. There were also cracks all around the circumference of the cylinder that formed the hydrophone mounting. Some of these cracks had paint on the surface, from which it may be deduced that they occurred during the welding operation. Most of the cracks, including those that were contaminated by paint, had a rough fibrous surface and lay about 1 mm below the plate surface. Such fractures are typical of the defect known as 'lamellar tearing' and are caused by a combination of shrinkage strain during cooling of the weld with low through-thickness ductility in the steel. This ductility was measured for the hydrophone fitting as between 1 and 7%, which indicates a very low resistance to lamellar tearing. The implication of these observations and tests is that for much, and probably most, of its life the fitting was only connected to the brace over part of the weld area. The result would have been to increase the level of strain around the fitting and to give a strain concentration effect in the regions where the fatigue crack initiated.

Various calculations have been made subsequently to determine the probable life expectancy of the brace D6. Assuming a sound weld between the hydrophone fitting and the brace, and using the data then available concerning wave frequency, it was estimated that the lifetime would be between 24 and 150 months. If the fitting had been completely separated, this estimate was reduced to between 10 and 54 months. The actual life was just over 40 months, so these estimates are reasonably close to the mark.

It would be reasonable to conclude that the most important factor leading to the premature failure of brace D6 was the use of low quality steel for the hydrophone fitting. A preliminary examination of one of the other fittings showed no surface cracking in the exterior weld and there was no evidence of incipient failure at other joints. Thus, although the design was suspect, defective material would seem to have been the reason why a potential for fatigue cracking developed into a catastrophic failure.

The historical perspective

When a mechanical failure gives rise to a disaster of such magnitude as that which befell the *Alexander L Kielland*, the adequacy of the design and control system is inevitably brought into question. In this case there were two organisations mainly responsible: the original designers, Institut Français du Pétrole and Neptune, and the classification society responsible for reviewing the design and carrying out inspection during the construction phase, Det Norske Veritas. It will be recalled that the design of Pentagone rigs 82–91, including No 89, *Alexander L Kielland*, was essentially the same, based on P 82, which was designed in 1970–71. P 89 was delivered in July 1976.

The 1970s were a period of considerable development in the understanding of how far, in quantitative terms, the presence of fillet-welded details affected the fatigue strength of steel. The fact that welding reduced the fatigue life had been known for a number of years and Gurney published a book on the subject in 1968.[12] In the early 1970s data on fatigue strength were gathered by the British Welding Institute and this resulted in proposals for design rules which appeared in 1976.[13] These proposals were incorporated in Part 10 of the British Standard for steel bridges BS 5400 in 1980. However, none of the classification societies had incorporated any provision for design against fatigue in their rules by 1976. There was therefore no reason to expect either Lloyd's Register (which was concerned with the original design) or Det Norske Veritas to have carried out a fatigue analysis. At the time it was generally assumed that the fatigue limit of carbon steel was about half the tensile strength, so any safety factor greater than two would take care of the problem.

Likewise there was no requirement for control of the through-thickness ductility of steel plate. Lamellar tearing had been encountered, but mostly in heavy plate fabrication and its potentially dire consequences in the welding of a detail such as the hydrophone mounting was certainly not understood at the time. It was only after the accident that it became normal practice to specify a minimum through-thickness ductility for steel used in critical joints; a typical minimum value in current practice is 20%.

The other design fault was that there was no redundancy in the structure; that is to say, if one major load-carrying member failed, others were overloaded and a collapse or partial collapse would be inevitable. At the time that the Pentagone rigs were developed it was already standard practice in some areas of engineering to protect against such an outcome;

for example, this was done in aircraft, where it was known as 'fail-safe' design. In some cases there is a built-in redundancy; for example, the hull plating of a ship provides an additional measure of support. Not surprisingly, the Commission of Inquiry recommended that semi-submersible rigs be designed to withstand the failure of a single member.

Escape craft

The difficulty and danger of launching lifeboats in heavy seas were undoubtedly some of the important factors leading to the heavy loss of life in the *Alexander L Kielland* accident. A further contribution was the difficulty of releasing the hooks which, in effect, tied the lifeboats to the wreck. It is vital that as soon as the boat is afloat the forward and aft hooks should be released simultaneously. The motion of the boat made this impossible in the case of the *Alexander L Kielland* because the hook could only be released when there was no tension, and when the boat rocked one hook was loose whilst the other was on load. The Commission of Inquiry could find no solution to this problem, because some time previously the release wire of a survival capsule had been operated prematurely and the capsule fell, killing three men. Subsequent to this tragedy, it was decided that hooks should not be releasable when under load and the Commission of Inquiry could not recommend any relaxation of this rule.

In other countries such a relaxation has been adopted and it is possible for those inside the boat to release the hooks simultaneously. A hydraulic interlock ensures that this can only be done when the boat is actually afloat. The Norwegian authorities have, however, opted for a much more radical solution: the free-fall lifeboat. The boat dives into the sea from a height of up to 30 m; there are no davits and no hooks, and once released the boat goes in the right direction, away from the wreck. Occupants of free-fall lifeboats lie prone on specially contoured beds and both body and head are restrained by straps. Where free-fall lifeboats are installed, personnel are trained in their use. This training includes at least one dive in a free-fall boat. To date the system works well during training, but it has yet to be tested in an emergency.

There were 212 men on board the *Alexander L Kielland* when the supporting column D collapsed. Of this complement 89 were rescued, and 123 lost their lives.

The Piper Alpha *disaster*

The Piper field, which produced both oil and gas, was at the time of the accident operated by the Occidental Group, and is located just over 100 miles north-east of Aberdeen, Scotland, in the North Sea. Figure 3.13 shows how the pipelines connected the three fixed units in the field, the gas compression platform MCP-01, and the two terminals, the oil terminal at Flotta in the Orkney Isles and the gas terminal at St Fergus in Scotland. Initially only oil was exported, gas which was surplus to platform requirements being flared, but in 1978 following governmental requirements for conservation, gas was exported to MCP-01 where it was mixed with gas from the Frigg gas field.

Figure 3.14 is a photograph of the *Piper Alpha* platform taken from the north-west, showing the accommodation with the helideck on top and the radio room on the far side of the helideck. The drilling derrick is at the rear. This rig provided means for drilling wells to the producing reservoir, together with process equipment to separate oil, water and gas and to separate gas (mainly methane) from condensate (mainly propane). Further processing of the gas and condensate was carried out on shore at the St Fergus terminal.

The jacket was a steel structure standing in water of depth 474 ft. There were decks at 20, 45, 68, 84, 107, 121 ft, then four levels of accommodation and the helideck at 174 ft. The production deck, which housed most of the processing equipment, was located at the 84 ft level, as outlined in Fig. 3.15.

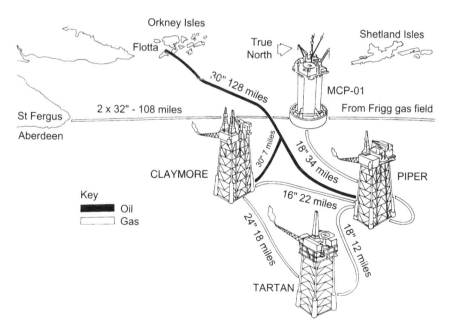

3.13 Pipeline connections in the Piper field in 1988.[14]

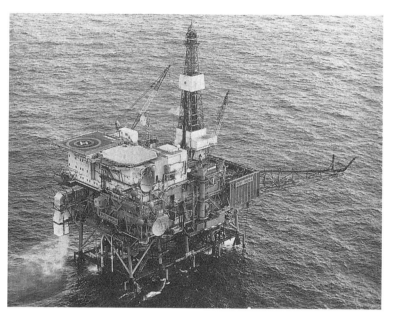

3.14 The *Piper Alpha* platform viewed from the north-west.[14]

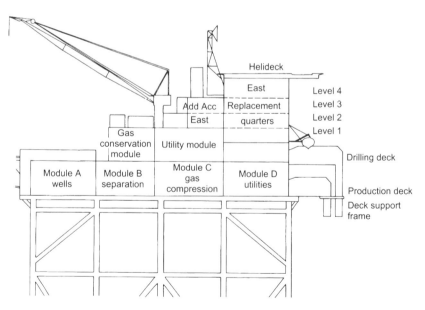

3.15 Layout of the topsides of the *Piper Alpha* platform.[14]

The area was divided into modules, each about 150 ft long, 50 ft wide and 24 ft high. On the left in Fig. 3.15 is A module, which contained the wellheads or 'Christmas trees' (so called because of their shape), of which there were 3 rows of 12.

The B module housed the two production separation vessels and one smaller test separator, together with the pumps for the main oil line. Module C contained the gas compressors with their associated scrubber vessels and coolers. There were three centrifugal and two reciprocating compressors. This is where the trouble started. D module was primarily for power generation. The gas conservation module, a later addition, was located as shown on the next level up; and below, on the 68 ft level, were the terminations of the gas lines from the Tartan and Claymore platforms and the gas line to the MCP-01 compression unit. This level contained the condensate injection pumps and the drum in which gas and condensate were separated. The diving area was also situated at the 68 ft level.

The control room was on a mezzanine floor, above the D module. In current practice, virtually all the operational functions of a process unit can be carried out in the control room, either by human beings or by computer. The *Piper Alpha* control room was an earlier type, where conditions in the plant were monitored and from which instructions to operators in the relevant module were issued. For example, if a high-level alarm showed up for a particular vessel, the control room operator telephoned the appropriate module operator to cut the flow to that vessel, which he did from a local control board.

The process unit

Figure 3.16 is a simplified process flow diagram for the unit as it was being operated at the time of the accident. The first step is primary separation, by gravity, of water, oil and gas. The water passed through a hydrocyclone to remove oil and was then discharged into the sea. Oil (which at that stage usually contained about 2% water) was pumped directly to Flotta. The gas, which consisted of a mixture of gaseous hydrocarbons, was compressed to 675 psi in three parallel centrifugal compressors, and then to 1735 psi by two parallel reciprocating compressors. In the operating mode in use at the time of the accident, the gas was then chilled by passing it through a Joule–Thomson expansion valve, where the pressure was reduced. The resulting fall in temperature caused higher hydrocarbons such as propane to condense, whilst lower hydrocarbons such as methane remained gaseous. These two phases were separated in a flash drum. The condensate was then compressed and injected into the main oil line, to be separated again at the terminal.

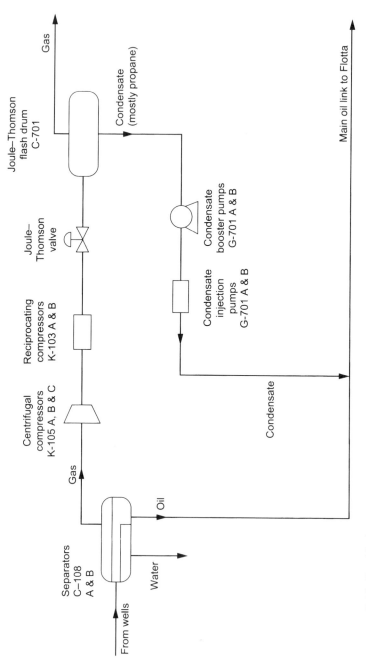

3.16 Simplified process flow diagram for *Piper Alpha*.

In the other operating mode, gas from the reciprocating compressors passed to the gas conservation module, where it first went through molecular sieve driers and then to a turbo-expander where the pressure dropped to about 635 psi. The condensate so formed went to a demethaniser tower where methane was stripped out and thence to the Joule–Thomson flash drum. Gas rejoined the original system downstream of the same flash driers.

Power

The main electrical supply came from two 24 000 kW generators driven by gas turbines. Normally the turbines were fired by fuel gas but they could alternatively operate with diesel fuel. In the event of a fall in gas pressure there was an automatic switch to diesel. However, this changeover was said to be less than 100% reliable. There was a completely separate power supply for drilling.

If the main supply failed, then a diesel-fired emergency generator came into operation. As backup, and to supply power to essential items whilst the emergency generator was running up to speed, there was a battery-powered supply.

6 July 1988

A contractor was in the course of calibrating some of the safety valves in the *Piper Alpha* process equipment. On this date, the last of the series, PSV504 on the condensate injection pump G701 A, which had already been shut down and electrically isolated in preparation for other maintenance work, was to be checked. As noted earlier, the condensate injection pumps were on the 68 ft level, but the relief valve was located above, in the corner of C module. The valve was removed in the early afternoon and a blind flange fitted in its place. It was duly tested and found satisfactory, but could not be replaced because there was no crane available. It was therefore agreed with the day-shift operators that the work should be completed on the following day.

At about 9.45 pm the same evening, after the night shift had taken over, the remaining condensate injection pump, G701 B, tripped out. This meant that the flow of condensate from the Joule–Thomson flash drum was arrested. The control room operator informed the operator in C module and at the same time the lead operator, who was in the control room, went down to try to restart the pump. Shortly after this, a high-level alarm showed up for the surge drum and the reciprocating compressors were put on recycle. It would then only be about half an hour before the gas supply to the main generators failed and the changeover to diesel fuel would be initiated. The operators were therefore under some pressure.

At this point the lead operator came back to the control room to report that the B compressor would not restart. The operators were, it would seem, unaware of the fact that the safety valve had been removed from the A compressor and they proceeded to cancel the 'permission to work' permit so that it could legitimately be reconnected to the electrical supply. The lead operator (who died in the disaster) then went back to the compressors.

Shortly after this, two of the centrifugal compressors tripped, and more or less at the same time a low-level gas alarm in C module was activated. Then things happened very quickly. A further set of gas alarms sounded in rapid succession, three low-level and one high-level, all in C module. The control room operator was trying to talk to the operator in C module above the noise of these alarms when the first explosion occurred. The time was 10.00 pm in the evening.

This was clearly a vapour cloud explosion, but the source of the vapour cannot be established with complete certainty. Nevertheless, the evidence assembled by Lord Cullen and the experts who conducted the public inquiry is very convincing. The lead operator, having signed off the permit to work on the G701 A pump returned to the 68 ft level, with the intention of arranging for the electric power to be reinstated. The first step in restarting the pump would be to open the valve on the suction (upstream) side and to admit condensate. From other evidence it is supposed that this action was taken and that the valve was opened for about 30 seconds. This would have had the effect of admitting condensate to the pump and to the relief valve line at a pressure of 670 pounds force per square inch absolute.

According to local practice, there were three levels to which the bolts fastening the blind flange to the relief valve piping could have been tightened: finger tight, hand tight (using a spanner) or flogged (using a flogging spanner). Tests subsequently showed that the second two levels of tightness would have made a leak-tight joint, but that a finger-tight joint would leak. Condensate escaping in this way would partially vaporise and would have provided a sufficiently large vapour cloud to account for the explosion. Other sources of vapour were considered to have been very much less probable.

Immediate effect of the explosion

Between C module and its neighbours, B and D, there were fire walls. These consisted of sheet steel bolted to a steel framework and insulated with mineral wool or other heat insulation material. The force of the explosion was sufficient to blow these walls out and cause fatal damage in the adjacent modules. In D module the main and emergency electrical systems and the control room were extensively damaged and air lines torn out. Thus all means of controlling the platform as a whole were lost in a fraction of a second. However, the system operated like the vacuum brakes on a vehicle; loss of air and power caused units to shut down and emergency valves to close. The flare continued to operate and would eventually have depressurised all or most of the units.

However, in B module the explosion had devastating effects. Disintegration of the fire wall provided flying debris which damaged pipework and caused a leak. This is thought to have occurred in the 4 in-line carrying condensate just upstream of the point where it joined the main oil line (see Fig. 3.15). This leak developed rapidly into a full-bore fracture, the condensate discharged with great force, causing a fireball and crude oil started to pour out of the main oil line, forming a large spreading fire. The cause of the full-bore fracture is not known, but experience shows that where there is a leak in a gas line due to a sudden local crack, an internal explosion can occur in the pipe, blowing it wide open. However this may be, the scene was set for a disastrous escalation.

The separators made a major source of fuel for the spreading fire: they contained about 50 tons of crude oil. Nevertheless, experts calculated that this would not be sufficient to account for the known degree of spread, and it seems likely that there was an additional source. There was an emergency shut-down valve in the main oil line which should have operated when power was lost. However, such valves do not always close fully, so a leak was possible. Pressure was maintained in the main oil line because oil production continued at both the Claymore and Tartan platforms. It was not until about an hour after the initial explosion that a shore-based manager instructed Claymore and Tartan to shut down and made arrangements for the terminal at Flotta to depressurise the line.

The fire had meantime spread down to the 68 ft level, where the three gas risers terminated. There were two import risers, one from Tartan and one from Claymore, and an export line to the compressor platform MCP-01. These were large-diameter high tensile steel lines; for example, the Tartan riser was 18 in in diameter with a 1 in thick wall, and the normal gas pressure was about 1700 psi. The risers and their associated pipelines contained large quantities of gas, such that to depressurise them by flaring off the contents took several days. In all cases the valve at the 68 ft level had closed after the initial explosion so those parts of the risers exposed to the fire were at full pressure.

At 10.20 pm the Tartan riser burst, causing a major explosion and engulfing the platform in a sudden and intense fire. The rupture was caused by the direct exposure of the pipe to fire, such that the strength of the steel was reduced. Under normal circumstances the riser would have been protected by a fire-water deluge, but the fire-water system had been disabled by the earlier explosion.

Half an hour later there was a third violent explosion, the vibration of which was felt a mile away. This explosion destroyed one of the rescue craft operating near the platform and killed all but one of the crew. It was almost certainly due to the rupture of the MCP-01 line.

At this stage the platform started to collapse. The jib and cap of the crane on the west side fell into the sea. Shortly after this there was a major structural failure in the centre of the platform. The drilling derrick fell across the pipe deck, which collapsed. At about this time, approximately an hour after the failure of the Tartan riser, there was a further major explosion which was probably due to rupture of the Claymore gas riser. The drill store, where a number of men had taken shelter, started to fall, forcing the men out and engulfing some in smoke and flames. The supports for the accommodation modules began to fail and one by one they fell into the sea, that on the north end overturning at 12.45 am. By this time the fire was mainly from some of the wells and from oil floating on the sea, the risers having disintegrated down to near sea level. Figure 3.17 shows

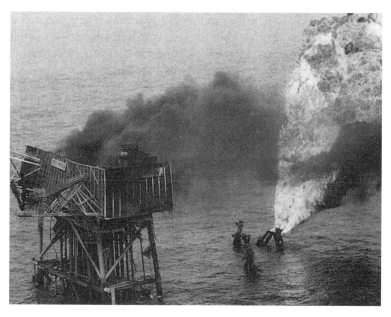

3.17 The remains of the *Piper Alpha* platform on the morning of 7 July. One of the risers is still burning (on the right of the picture). The black smoke is from the burning wells.[14]

the remains of the platform on the morning of 7 July, with flames still coming from one of the risers (presumably the MCP-01 line, which was 128 miles long – see Fig. 3.13). The black smoke is from the burning wells, seven of which were still flowing.

Evacuation and rescue

The emergency procedures for the rig required that the crew should muster in the accommodation area, where an emergency evacuation squad would direct parties to their respective lifeboats or to the helicopter. The whole operation was to be directed by the Offshore Installation Manager. In the event, these arrangements were completely set at nought by the failure of the public address system, such that no general directions could be given, and the rapid spread of the fire, which made access to the lifeboats impossible. It was clear to some of those on board at an early stage that smoke would make a helicopter landing difficult.

For those on the night shift there was no information at all and they had to make their own decisions. The divers, after recovering from the shock of the initial explosion, cast about for escape routes and found none, nor was there any way to get to their lifeboat. One of the team was working undersea; he was recovered and spent a short time in the decompression chamber. They then made their way on the 68 ft level to the north-west corner of the rig, which was fairly clear of smoke. In this location there were knotted ropes hanging over the edge of the platform and the men used these to climb down to the 20 ft level. Here they found rings attached to one of the platform legs and were able to climb down and step into one of the rescue boats. Others who were working on the 84 ft level went to the same point, including the two control room operators and 12 other men. Two of these fell off the ropes, and others were forced to jump into the sea from one level or the other.

Most of the drillers were able to go up to the accommodation level in accordance with the emergency procedure. There were already about 100 men in this area and eventually most of them made their way to the galley. Here the conditions were at first tolerable and there was hope either of a helicopter rescue or that the semi-submersible *Tharos*, which was nearby, would be able to get them off by a walkway. However, after the explosion of the Tartan riser at 10.20 pm many decided that the only way to be rescued was to get off the platform and found their way by various routes out of the accommodation. Seven went up on to the helideck and when the second major explosion occurred four of these jumped into the sea. They all survived, as did one other who jumped later off the helideck from 175 ft above the sea. Others went downwards and got off the platform into the sea by one means or another. Altogether there were 71 survivors. Sixty-three per cent of the night staff survived but only 13% of those off duty. When the accommodation units were recovered from the sea bed, 81 bodies were found inside. Altogether 165 of the 226 men on board lost their lives.

At the time of the disaster there were four vessels close to *Piper Alpha*. The standby was a converted trawler, the *Silver Pit*. It lay 250 m north-west of the platform. This vessel carried a fast rescue craft, a diesel-driven water-jet boat capable of 30 knots, which could carry three crew and up to 12 survivors. At 556 m was the *Tharos*. This was a semi-submersible that was equipped for fire-fighting, had a hospital with 22 beds, a fast rescue craft and a helicopter. She also had the means of launching a walkway onto a platform to evacuate crew. The *Maersk Cutter* was a supply vessel located about a mile from *Piper Alpha*. This had a fire monitor capable of discharging 10 000 tons of water per hour. The *Lowland Cavalier* lay 25 m off the south-west corner of the platform, engaged in trenching operations. Other vessels in the vicinity were the *Sandhaven*, a converted supply ship carrying a petrol-driven fast rescue craft, the *Loch Shuna* and the *Loch Carron*, also supply ships.

The *Tharos* started to move towards *Piper Alpha* immediately after the first explosion. Her helicopter was airborne at 10.11 pm but the pilot reported that the helideck was obscured by smoke. This helicopter was not equipped with a winch and it took no further part in the rescue operation. Preparations were then made to provide a cascade of water. This cascade came into action after some delay and provided a certain amount of protection against heat for the rescue boats and others. There was also an attempt to deploy the gangway. However, the landing position on the platform was shrouded in flame and smoke and the attempt was abandoned. Eventually when the MCP-01 riser exploded, *Tharos* was partly enveloped by the fireball and was drawn back by 100 m. Meantime, the *Maersk Cutter* had been directing water jets at the drill floor and continued to do so until shortly after midnight.

Fast rescue craft had been launched from a number of vessels and these were mainly responsible for picking up survivors. The first was from the *Silver Pit*, and it was this boat that picked up the divers, amongst others. It carried on working until after midnight, when the hull and engine were damaged by a further explosion. Its occupants were rescued by the *Maersk Cutter*. The fast rescue boat from the *Sandhaven* had picked up four men from the south-west corner of the platform when the MCP-01 riser ruptured. The explosion and fireball destroyed the boat. Two of the crew and all those that had been rescued were killed.

Of the 61 survivors, 37 reached the *Silver Pit*, 29 having been picked up by the rescue boat and the remainder by the vessel itself. Others were taken by rescue boats to the *Tharos* or were picked up directly by this vessel or the *Maersk Cutter*. No lifeboats were launched from *Piper Alpha* and there were no helicopter rescues.

Essential features of the Piper Alpha *disaster*

The series of explosions and fires on board *Piper Alpha* arose because an operator was attempting to start up a condensate compressor and as a preliminary step, pressurised the pump and the relief valve line. He was aware that the pump had been electrically isolated preparatory to maintenance work but (it is virtually certain) did not know that the safety valve had been removed for calibration and had not been replaced. The safety valve was located at a higher platform level than the compressor and was not visible from the compressor itself. Pressurising the pump caused a leak of condensate leading to a vapour cloud explosion which destroyed all means of control on the platform and initiated a major fire, fuelled by crude oil from the separators and also possibly from the main oil line. As a result of the loss of power, all emergency shutdown valves closed, including those on the import and export gas risers. These shutdown valves were located at the platform level which was seriously affected by the fire. The piping was weakened by heating in the fire, and three of the risers burst one after the other. Because these risers were connected to lengthy pipelines (in one case 128 miles long) and because the gas was under high pressure, there was an intense fire that persisted for a long time and eventually destroyed the platform.

The high loss of life was due eventually to two factors: first, there was no means of escaping the potentially deadly effects of smoke and secondly, there was no means of access to lifeboats or other orderly means of escape. Only those who were bold enough to jump into the sea or lucky enough to be near an easy escape route survived.

The South Pass 60 *Platform 'B' fire*

In March 1989, less than a year after the *Piper Alpha* catastrophe, there was a similar type of accident in the Mexican Gulf off the coast of Louisiana. Platforms in the Gulf are normally much smaller than those in the North Sea. The unit in question had 11 risers, one carrying oil, one condensate and the remainder gas. On 19 March a contractor's crew were cutting an 18 in gas riser in preparation for installing a pig trap. They had just penetrated the pipe wall when condensate started to spray out. The vapour was ignited by nearby machinery and a considerable fire ensued, the gas pressure in the riser being 1000 psi. The emergency shutdown system came into operation and, in particular, valves on all the other risers closed. As in the case of *Piper Alpha* these valves were above the source of the fire, and eventually six of the risers burst and the explosions and fires destroyed the platform, which finished up in much the same condition as *Piper Alpha*. Not only were the mechanics of this accident similar, but the action which initiated it resulted from the same human cause: a failure of communication, and in particular, a failure to plan the piping modifications so that they would be safe and so that all concerned were aware of potential hazards.

Seven men died as a result of this disaster. The US task group that was given the job of reviewing the *Piper Alpha* and the *South Pass 60* incidents concluded that if the workforce on *South Pass* had been of similar size, then the casualties could have been as high as those on *Piper Alpha*.[15]

Protecting the gas risers

The problem about gas is its compressibility. The compressibility of liquids is small, so that a pipeline carrying liquid hydrocarbons can be depressurised by drawing off a small fraction of its total content. This can be accomplished in a short space of time. To depressurise a gas line operating at 3000 psi (not an uncommon pressure in offshore work) by flaring to atmosphere could require the burning of about 20 times the volume of the pipeline, which would take a long time. Likewise, a fire following a full-bore rupture persists for a period long enough to cause structural collapse of the surrounding steelwork.

One way of reducing the risk of failure due to an external fire is to insulate the riser. This was done in the case of one of the Ekofisk platforms situated in the Norwegian section of the North Sea, but corrosion occurred under the insulation and eventually the pipe leaked and there was a fire. It was during the evacuation of this platform that the hooks of a lifeboat were accidentally released, killing three men. This was the incident that caused the Norwegian authorities to specify the type of hook that gave such trouble to those trying to launch lifeboats when the *Alexander L Kielland* was sinking – not the first time that a safety prescription has defeated the intention of its authors. Regardless of its other consequences, the Ekofisk fire has more or less ruled out insulation as a means of protecting risers.

The alternative safety measure is to locate an emergency shutdown valve on the sea bed below the platform. Figure 3.18 shows the location of such a valve diagrammatically. In the North Sea these subsea valves are often large and very costly pieces of equipment and their installation is also a costly operation. Nevertheless, after the loss of the *Piper Alpha*, operating companies set about fitting such valves on a considerable scale. The

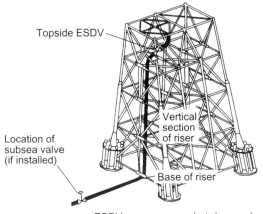

Topside ESDV

Vertical
section
of riser

Location of
subsea valve
(if installed)

Base of riser

ESDV = emergency shut-down valve

3.18 Diagram showing typical location of a subsea emergency shutdown valve
for a gas riser.[16,17]

improvement in safety will be self-evident; the relatively short length of line
downstream of the subsea valve could, in an emergency, be depressurised
in a short time via the normal flare system. Of course not all risers need
to be treated in this way and each case has to be treated on its merits.

The response of regulating bodies and operating companies

At the time of the *Piper Alpha* disaster, offshore safety in the British sector
of the North Sea was the responsibility of the Department of Energy. A
commission of inquiry into the disaster was set up under the chairmanship
of Lord Cullen and this reported in October 1990. Its recommendations
were numerous, but the core requirement was that companies operating
in the British sector should prepare a 'Safety Case'. This document is
essentially a review of the company's safety procedures and is intended to
assure the regulatory body that the safety objectives stated in the report of
the inquiry commission have been met. The only hardware requirement is
that a temporary safe haven, usually the accommodation block, where
occupants would be protected for a period of, say, two hours should be
provided. Otherwise, the necessary measures would be proposed by the
operating company and agreed with the regulatory body, intended to be a
special section of the Health and Safety Executive. There is no requirement
for subsea isolation valves.

Safety on the US continental shelf is regulated by the Minerals
Management Service of the Department of the Interior. A task force was

set up to review regulations in the light of the *Piper Alpha* and *Southpass 60* 'B' disasters. There was in place a regulation requiring that out-of-service devices be identified or 'flagged'. It was recommended that such identification be extended to pumps and flow control valves upstream of the flagged equipment, that personnel with the authority to remove flags be identified, and that all workers on platforms be informed of out-of-service equipment, repair activities and safety concerns. Various other detailed recommendations were made regarding fire-water pumps and providing a safe haven (more or less on the same lines as the British recommendations). They further set in hand a consultative review of the possibility of installing subsea valves. Figure 3.19 is an outline sketch of a large off shore fixed platform incorporating some of the lessons learnt from the *Piper Alpha* disaster.

Level 1 Export equipment area
Level 2 Separation and manifolds
Level 3 Gas compression and final separation
Level 4 LNG chillers and gas compression coolers

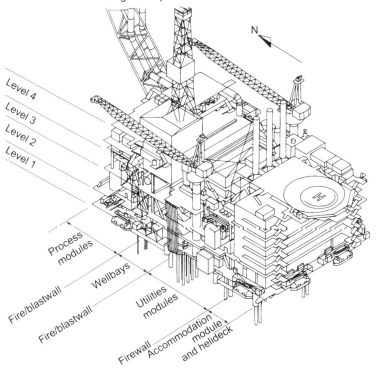

3.19 Diagram of the topsides of the *Tiffany* platform, incorporating safety features.[18]

Catastrophes involving air travel

The Comet I aircraft failures

These early jet aircraft first took off a long time ago and the company that made them no longer exists. Nevertheless, there were important technical lessons to be learnt from their loss, lessons that are not always fully understood today, so the history of the disasters is still worthy of study. Fortunately, a very lucid account of the accidents was provided by the court of inquiry which met under the chairmanship of Lord Cohen.[19]

Comets were built by the de Havilland Aircraft Company and the engines were supplied by a subsidiary, the de Havilland Engine Company. De Havilland was founded immediately after the First World War by Captain Geoffrey de Havilland. It manufactured civil aircraft, which in the early days were biplanes powered by a single engine. They were numbered successively, the 1920 version DH 16, 1924 DH 34 and so on. Comet was DH 106. During the Second World War the entire output of the company consisted of military planes, but in 1945 it reverted to the civil field. The engine company had experience with gas turbines, so it was decided to take a bold step and design a jet airliner. At that time communications within the British Empire offered a lucrative trade: flights were long, and a jet aircraft could halve the flight time.

Design work on the prototype started in September 1946. At the beginning of the following year the British Overseas Aircraft Corporation (BOAC) and the Government Ministry concerned signed a contract for the purchase of Comet aircraft and this enabled de Havilland to go ahead with production. Two prototypes were delivered in 1951 and BOAC started proving flights, having been issued with temporary certificates of airworthiness. By 1952 a full airworthiness certificate was obtained and a passenger service was started, the first flight being to Johannesburg in South Africa.

Design

Turbo-jet engines consume fuel at a much lower rate at high altitudes than they do lower down. For this reason it was necessary that the Comet should be designed to fly at 35 000 ft or more. For the comfort of passengers and crew it was therefore necessary to pressurise the cabin. An excess pressure P (difference between internal and external pressure) of $8\frac{1}{4}$ psi was required, 50% higher than that of any other aircraft operating at the time. Initially the design was based on static loading. The International Civil Aviation Organisation and also the British airworthiness authority (the Air

Registration Board), required that the maximum working stress should be less than half the ultimate strength of the material, and that the cabin should show no permanent deformation at an internal pressure excess of $1\frac{1}{3}P$. De Havilland went further and used a design stress of $\frac{2}{5}$ ultimate strength and a test pressure of $2P$. This, they considered, would take care of any fatigue problems. They were also concerned to have a good margin of safety against the failure of individual windows, doors and hatches, with good reason because sudden depressurisation can cause death or injury to passengers and crew. Two test sections of cabin were built. The first part extended from the nose to the front spar of the wing, where it was sealed to a steel bulkhead. The second part extended 24 ft from just in front of the wing to a small distance aft of the wing. Both included typical windows, hatches and doors. These test sections were subjected to 30 applications of pressure of between P and $2P$, and 200 pressurisations of just over P. Such tests were not intended to check the fatigue resistance, but were simply repeated static tests. Fatigue tests were, however, carried out on the wings, because fatigue cracking had been found in the wings of certain transport aircraft some time previously.

In 1952 it became evident from experience with military aircraft that fatigue failure could also occur as the result of repeated pressurisation of the cabin. The Air Registration Board therefore proposed that in addition to the static test, there should be a repeated loading test of 15 000 cycles at a pressure of $1\frac{1}{4}P$. In the middle of 1953 de Havilland decided that it was necessary to carry out such tests on the Comet cabin. They used the test section that ran from the nose to the wing and subjected this to repeated pressurisations at the working pressure P, in addition to the static pressure tests that were done previously. The repeated loading test was discontinued when a crack, which originated at a defect in the skin, appeared near the corner of a window. By this time the pressure had been applied 18 000 times and all concerned felt assured of the safety of the cabin.

The disaster

There had been a series of take-off incidents with the Comet in the early days, which culminated in a crash and fire at Karachi airport. These were originally put down to pilot error but further investigation showed that they were due to the wing section, and the problem was overcome by making some modifications. Then in May 1953 a Comet in flight from Calcutta to Karachi broke up in the air during a violent storm. On examining the wreckage it was found that the tail portion had broken away. It was concluded that in trying to counter the severe turbulence associated with the storm, the pilot had imposed loads that the airframe could not withstand. The earlier Comets were fitted with power-assisted controls so that it was possible to apply considerable force without being aware of the fact. Subsequently a synthetic resistance was applied to such controls which enabled the pilot to judge how much force he was applying to control surfaces.

Following these modifications all went well until January 1954, when Comet G-ALYP took off from Rome airport on a flight to London. At about 9.50 am that morning another BOAC aircraft received a message from the Comet: 'George How Jig from George Yoke Peter did you get my' – at which point the message broke off abruptly. At this time the Comet would have been at about 27 000 ft and still climbing. Ten minutes later farmers on the island of Elba saw aircraft wreckage, some of which was on fire, fall into the sea. The harbourmaster at Portoferraio was informed and he very promptly assembled a search and rescue team and set off for the area where the wreckage had been seen. Fifteen bodies, some mailbags and some floating wreckage were recovered. At the time of the accident, the aircraft was carrying 29 passengers and six crew, all of whom were killed.

It was evidently not a repeat of the Calcutta incident because the weather on this occasion was clear with little turbulence. The water was 400–600 ft in depth so salvage was possible, and the British Navy was given the job of recovering as much material as possible. Vessels were fitted with grabs and heavy lifting gear. They used a television camera underwater (the first time television had been employed in such an operation) to locate the wreckage. After about three weeks' search the remains were located and a fair proportion was recovered.

In the meantime all Comet flights had been suspended and a committee of investigation had been set up under the chairmanship of Mr Abell of BOAC. By that time the fatigue test on the wings had generated a few cracks so that it was decided to strengthen the affected parts. The possibility of fatigue cracking of the cabin was discounted in view of the tests at de Havilland and the committee took the view that fire was the most likely cause of the accident. Following this conclusion there was no reason why services should not be resumed, and so they restarted on 23 March 1954.

On 8 April of the same year a Comet took off from Rome airport on a flight to Cairo. Just over half an hour later, when the aircraft would have been close to or at its cruising height, radio contact was lost. The following day bodies and wreckage were recovered from the sea off the Italian coast near Naples. It was obvious at once that the design of the aircraft was seriously flawed and it was grounded again, this time permanently.

The similarity of the two accidents, in particular the fact that they had apparently broken up just before reaching cruising altitude, suggested that the cabin might have exploded because of the presence (against previous evidence) of fatigue cracks. Accordingly, a water tank large enough to contain a complete aircraft was constructed and used to carry out fatigue tests on one of the Comets from the BOAC fleet. These tests were conducted with the cabin completely submerged so that there was no additional stress imposed by the weight of the water. The cycle consisted of pressurisation up to the normal excess of $8\frac{1}{4}$ psi, combined with loading of the wings to simulate flight conditions. Every 1000 cycles a pressure of 11 psi was applied. The aircraft used in this test had made 1230 pressurised flights and its cabin failed after 1830 pressurisations in the tank, making a total of 3060. The first service failure, at Elba, occurred after 1290 flights, and the second after 900 flights. At the time the court of inquiry considered that the shorter life of the service aircraft was due to their exposure to a multitude of additional stresses when airborne, and this conclusion seems reasonable in retrospect.

Two further steps were taken at this stage. Strain-gauge measurements were made of the stress at the corner of the windows, and these showed that the highest stress, at the edge of the skin near the corner, was in the region of 40 000 psi, about twice the figure which had been calculated by de Havilland, and about two-thirds of the ultimate tensile strength of the material. The figure of 40 000 psi was not in itself very significant but it indicated a high general level of stress in the vicinity. Most of the fatigue cracks in later tests originated at the rivet holes, which cause a localised increase in stress up to a factor of three.

The second step was to recover more of the wreckage, by trawling along the line of flight in the direction of Rome airport. This produced further sections of the wing which showed paint marks, indicating that it had been struck by fragments of the cabin whilst in flight. It also produced a portion of the cabin that had originally been located above the wing, and which contained two windows. By examining the fracture surfaces the investigators were able to pinpoint the probable origin of the failure as a fatigue crack at the corner of one of the windows (Fig. 3.20). When this crack had propagated to a critical length the centre portion of the cabin exploded, the probable lines of separation being as shown in Fig. 3.21.

Further testing

A second series of fatigue tests were made on the fuselage of another Comet I aircraft, using the same tank but applying an internal pressure that alternated from zero to $8\frac{1}{4}$ psi only.[20] There was no additional loading of the structures. The results of those tests indicate very clearly the way in which fatigue cracks and the final catastrophic failure occurred.

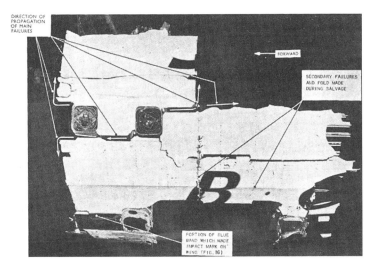

DIRECTION OF
PROPAGATION
OF MAIN
FAILURES

FORWARD

SECONDARY FAILURES
AND FOLD MADE
DURING SALVAGE

PORTION OF BLUE
BAND WHICH MADE
IMPACT MARK ON
WING (FIG. 16)

3.20 Wreckage of part of the cabin of Comet G-ALYP, pieced together to show the direction of fracture propagation. This section was immediately above the wing.

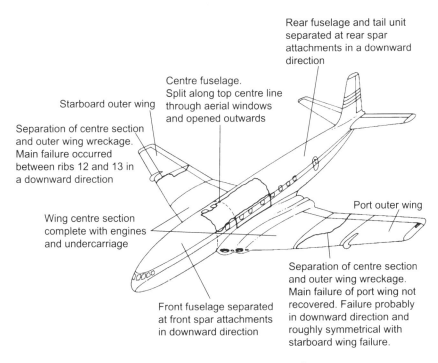

Rear fuselage and tail unit separated at rear spar attachments in a downward direction

Centre fuselage.
Split along top centre line through aerial windows and opened outwards

Starboard outer wing

Separation of centre section and outer wing wreckage. Main failure occurred between ribs 12 and 13 in a downward direction

Port outer wing

Wing centre section complete with engines and undercarriage

Separation of centre section and outer wing wreckage. Main failure of port wing not recovered. Failure probably in downward direction and roughly symmetrical with starboard wing failure.

Front fuselage separated at front spar attachments in downward direction

3.21 Location of main failures in Comet G-ALYP.[19]

Table 3.3 Materials used in cabin structure of Comet I aircraft

(a) Composition, % by mass

Copper	3.5–4.8
Iron	less than 1.0
Silicon	less than 1.5
Magnesium	less than 1.0
Manganese	less than 1.2
Titanium	less than 0.3

(b) Mechanical properties (minimum)

	0.1% proof stress		Ultimate stress		Elongation (%)
	tons/sq in	psi	tons/sq in	psi	
DTD 610	14	31360	24	53760	12
DTD 546B	20	44800	26	58240	8

The materials used for the cabin structure are detailed in Table 3.3. The alloy composition was similar to that currently designated as 2024; a high-strength copper/magnesium/manganese/silicon alloy, heat-treated to give two different strength levels. The higher tensile material was used for the skin and the lower tensile for circumferential frames and window frames.

The de Havilland fatigue tests

It will be recalled that de Havilland had carried out fatigue tests on a section of the fore part of the cabin and that this withstood 18 000 applications of the working pressure before a fatigue crack appeared. However, the same test section had previously been subject to a number of overpressure tests; 30 applications of between working pressure and twice working pressure. The effect of such overpressure is to cause regions of stress concentration to yield plastically, such that when the pressure is removed they are in a state of compressive stress. When subsequently these same regions are loaded in tension, the strain only becomes tensile after the initial compressive strain has been overcome. Therefore, in a pulsating tensile condition, the tensile part of the loading cycle is reduced. Since it is primarily tensile loading that causes fatigue damage, the fatigue life is increased; in this case about threefold. The beneficial effect of the initial overpressure test is applicable to those areas, in this instance around the outer row of rivet holes, at the corners of the windows, that are most likely to initiate cracks under fatigue loading conditions.

The lesson is that fatigue testing of a structure (or any other test for that matter) should reproduce as precisely as possible the pattern of loading that is to be found in service and that testing of pre-strained samples is not valid.

The explosion

The Comet I disasters occurred at a time when the discipline of fracture mechanics was under development in the USA, for example at the Naval Research Laboratory in Washington, DC, under the leadership of G R Irvine. A A Wells was seconded to the Naval Research Laboratory during that period and later returned to the British Welding Research Association (now TWI) to conduct some tests on the aluminium alloys used for the construction of the Comet.

The tests were made on samples of sheet containing a central slot, the ends of which were sharpened by loading for a short period in a fatigue testing machine. Theory predicts that if a plate or sheet of brittle material containing a crack of length a is exposed to a tensile stress σ, then the crack will start to propagate when the quantity $\sigma^2 a$ rises to a critical value. The tests showed this relationship to be true for precipitation-hardened aluminium alloys and indicated that the critical value of $\sigma^2 a$ for DTD 546B would be 250 inch-(tons/square inch)^2 (equivalent to $39\,\mathrm{MN/m^{3/2}}$, see Appendix 2). The stress in the skin of the Comet caused by pressurisation alone was about 6.3 tons/square inch so the calculated critical crack length for catastrophic failure would have been $250/(6.3)^2 = 6.3\,\mathrm{in}$. The actual critical length determined in the second series of tank tests was indeed about 6 in.

Once an unstable crack initiates it will propagate at very high speed. In steel speeds of thousands of feet per second have been measured. The failure of the Comet fuselage therefore could have been, for all practical purposes, instantaneous, and the deaths of passengers and crew would probably have occurred within a fraction of a second.

The final phase

De Havilland eventually succeeded in producing a sound design and the Comet IV went into service in the late 1950s. It was the first jet aircraft to go into regular passenger service across the Atlantic. But by this time the Boeing Corporation had developed a jet aircraft (the Boeing 707) which had a higher capacity and greater range than the Comet, and this came into use shortly afterwards. So in the end, the Comet was grounded not by technical problems, but because its performance was not good enough.

Postscript

In a television programme presented in 2003, it was stated that during the construction of the Comet I aircraft, the works manager of de Havilland reported that he could not produce a satisfactory araldite bonded joint between the hull and the window reinforcing frames and requested permission to use rivets at the corners. This was agreed. Photographs of the wreck in this region show displacements that are, indeed, consistent with a failure of, or lack of, adhesive bonding in this area. There is good reason to suppose that if the frames had been securely bonded, then the aircraft would not have exploded. This is an example where relaxing specifications for the sake of expediency in manufacture led to catastrophe; one which should provide a lesson for all engineers.

British airships: the R 101

Airships, in hindsight, never had much chance of success. Their basic defect was that even using the lightest gas, hydrogen, the achievable lift was relatively small, and it diminished with height, such that the machines were forced to travel at about 1000–2000 ft, an altitude at which they were highly vulnerable to weather. The optimum cruising speed was low, typically 50–60 mph. Between the two world wars, though, these problems were outweighed by the potential advantage of range, which was measured in thousands of miles, and a passenger capacity that was potentially many times that of contemporary aircraft. Thus, it was possible to think about providing round-the-world passenger services with comfort and leg-room, and with journey times reduced from weeks to days.

Airships were flown in France in the middle of the nineteenth century, but the first practical passenger-carrying craft was produced by Count Ferdinand von Zeppelin, who developed the idea of setting a row of spherical gas bags in a tubular steel framework, the whole being powered by internal combustion engines driving propellers, suspended below the framework. Prior to and immediately after the First World War, a German company ran a large number of pleasure fights in Zeppelins without a single casualty although during the war it was otherwise. Zeppelins were employed to bomb London but the losses were so high that their use was abandoned in 1917 in favour of heavier-than-air craft. In the 1920s and 1930s Zeppelins operated on long-distance flights, including a scheduled service between Europe and South America. In the early years of the twentieth century, therefore, airships seemed to have a bright future.

In England airships had a shaky start. The first was designed by Vickers Limited on the lines of a light submarine. Unfortunately, it turned out to be over heavy, and to lighten it, the keel was removed. As a result it broke its back while being towed out into open water. Subsequent developments were all land-based, the design relying heavily on information obtained, in one way or another, about Zeppelins. There was a success, the R 34, which flew to New York and back in 1919, and a catastrophe, the R 38, which broke up in the air during a demonstration flight. Then, in 1924, it was decided to proceed with the construction of two large ships, the R 100 and R 101, which would pioneer regular passenger services to India.

An initial step was the construction of mooring masts. These were towers about 200 ft in height to which the aircraft was attached. Figure 3.22 is a sketch of the layout at the top of the tower. The airship was towed to the mast by a cable powered by a stationary engine and was steadied by side guys. Passengers came up by lift and boarded by means of the ramp shown.

Mooring masts were built at the Royal Aircraft Works in Cardington, Bedford, England, in Ottawa, Canada, in Karachi (then India) and in Ismailia, Egypt, which was the intended intermediate stop on the India route. Between flights the airships were housed in sheds, into and out of which they were moved by large gangs of men. If the crew were sufficiently skilled, a mooring mast was not essential. When the Graf Zeppelin visited

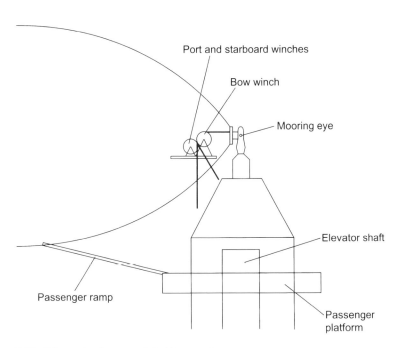

3.22 Schematic diagram of airship mooring mast.

Cardington, it was manœuvred within a few feet of the ground and held by guys whilst passengers disembarked and embarked using a gangway.

The Ministry specifications for the R 100 and R 101 required that the gasbag capacity be five million cubic feet, and that the ships be capable of carrying 100 passengers to India with one refuelling stop in Egypt. They were to be capable of flying at 70 miles per hour and to have a speed of at least 63 miles per hour average over a 48-hour period. One ship was to be built under contract by Vickers Ltd, and the other by the government establishment at Cardington. This inept arrangement established two design and construction teams, one of which (Vickers) was working for and reporting to the other (the government establishment at Cardington): inevitably there was friction. It happened that one of the designers of the Vickers airship, the R 100, was the novelist Nevil Shute (in real life Nevil Shute Norway) and he has left a vivid account of this rivalry.[21] At a later date Peter Masefield, who advised the British Government about the possibility of airship development after the Second World War, wrote a very detailed history of the other craft, the R 101.[22] The subject has therefore been well documented.

A major handicap to the whole project was the belief, firmly held by engineers in the Air Ministry, that petrol engines were unsafe under tropical conditions. It was thought that the low flash point of gasoline meant that they would explode or catch fire in a hot climate. Therefore, the Cardington team opted for diesel engines and as a result suffered a weight penalty of 7 tons. Since Vickers used petrol engines, the R 100 was considered unsuitable for the India route and was scheduled to go to Canada instead.

In other respects the general arrangement of the two ships was rather similar. Both had passenger and crew accommodation inboard, located just above the control car. On R 100 the accommodation was on three decks, on R 101 it was on two. The outline of R 101 is shown in Fig. 3.23 and details of the accommodation are given in Fig. 3.24. The lounge of the R 100 is shown in Fig. 3.25.

There was, however, a very important difference between the two airships. Table 3.4 shows the available lift of the two ships on the date of their first flight (both in 1929) compared with 1924 Ministry requirements. R 100 was 10 tons short, but it could still have carried (in theory at least) about 40 passengers to India, whereas R 101 was not capable of making the trip even without passengers. So it was decided that R 101 would be modified by inserting two extra bags, thereby increasing the lift by about 10 tons. R 100 meantime carried out its initial test flights, which were passed satisfactorily. There were, however, problems with the outer cover which required modification.

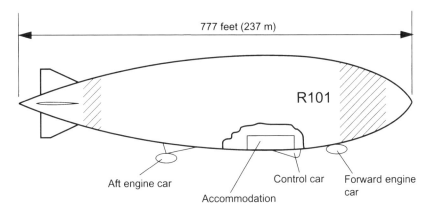

3.23 Outline sketch of airship R 101. The cross-hatching indicates areas of the outer cover that were not replaced during the 1930 refit.

The outer cover was an unending problem with airships. It consisted of cotton or linen cloth which was stretched over the framework of girders, and then treated with dope. This substance, also used at that time for heavier-than-air machines, consisted of a solution of cellulose derivatives such as cellulose acetate in a volatile liquid, and it had the effect, it was hoped, of increasing the strength of the cloth. However, tears were quite frequent and repairs were required during and between flights. Covers often leaked in a rainstorm and the gasbags became soaked. Alternative materials were Duralumin or stainless steel, but both were considered to be too heavy. No solution had been found to this problem when airships were finally grounded.

By early 1930, political problems had become acute. The programme was in its sixth year and there were no visible results, except for a round-Britain tour by R 100. An Imperial Conference was due to begin in September 1930 and it was planned that the Secretary of State for Air, Lord Thomson, should present an opening paper on the progress of imperial communications. It was intended that in October the initial flight to India would be made, with Lord Thomson on board, and that he would return in triumph to present a follow-up paper to the conference.

As a start R 100 was, after many delays, despatched to Canada at the end of July. Major G H Scott, a flyer of the old, press-on-regardless school, was in charge. The trip was a success in that the airship returned to Cardington in one piece. However, in Canada they had encountered a thunderstorm, and instead of avoiding it, Major Scott ordered the helmsman to go straight through. This smashed a lot of crockery and

Windows

Promenade deck

Cabins

Lounge

Dining room

Promenade deck

Windows

Upper deck

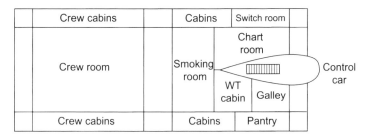

Crew cabins		Cabins	Switch room
Crew room	Smoking room	Chart room	Control car
		WT cabin	Galley
Crew cabins		Cabins	Pantry

Lower deck

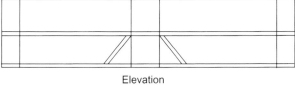

Elevation

3.24 Interior layout of airship R 101.

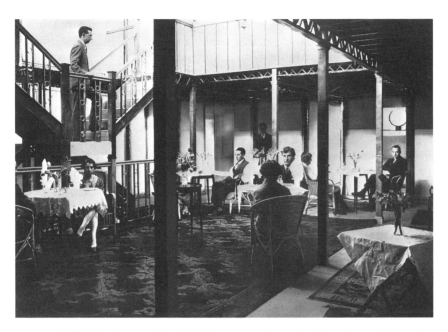

3.25 The lounge of the R 100. The person descending the stairway is the author Nevil Shute Norway.

Table 3.4 Airship weights: UK 1924 programme

Item	Air ministry specification 1924	Airship at the time of first flight	
		R 100	R 101
Volumetric capacity, cubic feet	5 million	5.156 million	4.894 million
Standard gross lift, tons	151.8	156.5	148.6
Fixed weight, tons	90.0	105.5	113.6
Disposable lift, tons	61.8	51.0	35.0
Ship prepared for service, with crew, stores and equipment, tons	110.0	125.5	133.6
Lift available for fuel and payload, tons	41.8	31.0	15.0
Fuel for journey to Egypt, tons	25.0	25.0	25.0
Lift available for payload, tons	16.8	6.0	Nil
Allowance for passengers (350 lb (159 kg) each), tons (number)	15.6 (100)	6.0 (38)	Nil
Allowance for mail, etc, tons	1.2	Nil	Nil

damaged the cover, which required extensive repairs. On the return journey across the Atlantic the ship ran into a rainstorm and water poured into the accommodation area, putting both heating and cooking equipment out of commission. Fortunately, the passengers and crew had been issued with fleece-lined flying suits. This was the twelfth and fastest crossing of the Atlantic by an airship. R 100 was then manhandled into a shed and never flew again.

In the meantime, work was proceeding on the lengthening of R 101. In addition to this major refit, most of the outer cover had been replaced. The original material had been doped before it was fitted, and in 1929 was found to be in poor condition. This was thought to be due to the predoping, so the new cover was doped *in situ*. Two parts of the cover that had previously been treated in this way (cross-hatched in Fig. 3.23) were not replaced. Then on 24 September, just before the ship was due to be handed over to the flying staff, it was found that rubber solution had been used to attach patches and reinforcing strips to the old cover aft of the nose. Rubber solution applied over dope rots the cloth, but it was now too late for any replacement. So further reinforcing strips were stuck over the affected areas with red dope, which is a compatible adhesive. The ship was passed by the inspectors on 27 September, but could not be brought out of the shed until 1 October because of bad weather. Since the scheduled departure date for India was 4 October, the duration of the test flight was reduced to 24 hours from 48 hours. This flight took place during the night of 1–2 October in clear weather with no turbulence. The flight instructions for the test required that the airship should run at full power from all five engines for at least 5 minutes. In the event an oil cooler failed on one of the engines and could not be replaced. Therefore the full power test was never done.

The disaster

Departure time was set for 18.30 pm Greenwich Mean Time on Saturday, 4 October, so that the ship would arrive at Ismailia, Egypt, in the early evening when, in the relatively cool conditions, there would be maximum lift. The weather forecast issued that afternoon predicted moderate wind over northern France, with light winds and clear weather over southern France and the Mediterranean. The conditions appeared to be promising; however, from the time the ship slipped its moorings they started to deteriorate. At first she was flown on a circular course such that it would have been possible to return to the mast (Fig. 3.26). Then, after about three-quarters of an hour of flying, it was finally decided to proceed south *en route* to Egypt.

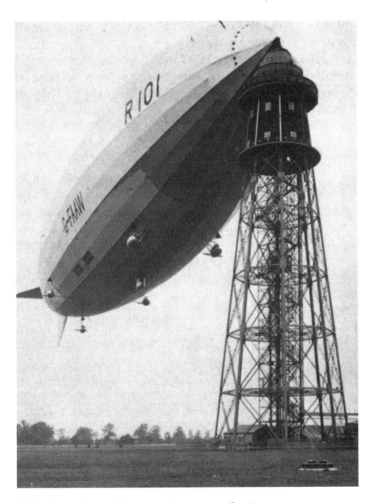

3.26 The airship R 101 leaving the mast at Cardington.

By this time it was raining and there was a strong south-westerly wind, with a cloud-base at 1500 ft. The cruising speed was 62 mph and height 1200 ft. Owing to the head wind component, however, the ground speed was just below 30 mph. Half an hour before midnight the airship crossed the French coast and rose to 1500 ft to clear the higher ground. The weather was getting worse, with heavy rain, turbulence and gusts of up to 50 mph.

At 2 am on 5 October the morning watch took over (airships adhered to naval traditions). The second officer, Maurice Steff, was in command in the control car with chief coxswain George Hunt. At 2.07 am, after the ship had passed over Beauvais, Hunt came up into the chart room from the control car and told a member of the crew to go forward and release ballast.

Then he called out 'we're down lads' (the chief electrician, Arthur Disley, who was in the switch room, heard this) and ran off, no doubt to warn the crew. At the same moment the ship lurched into a nose-down attitude and dived. After about a minute she came back on an even keel and a telegraph message was sent from the control car to reduce speed. Then after a few seconds the airship dived again and hit the ground just about 10 minutes after the start of the first dive. Within seconds a fierce fire broke out, consuming everything except the broken metal skeleton as evidenced in Fig. 3.27.

Harry L Leach, a foreman engineer, had gone to the smoking room (which was fire insulated) for a cigarette before turning in. When the ship levelled out he had time to pick himself up and replace some glasses and a soda-water siphon on the table. Then came the crash: the door of the smoking room flew open and he could see the flames surrounding the control car. Then the upper passenger deck collapsed but was supported at a height of about 3 ft by the room's furniture. At the same time a bulkhead fell out and he was able to crawl into the hull and thence on to the ground.

In number 5 after engine car Joe Binks was just taking over (a few minutes late) from engineer A V Bell. When the ship went into its second dive the engine telegraph pointer moved to 'slow' and Bell throttled down accordingly. Then came the crash, explosions and fire burning all around. The bottom of the car had been damaged and flames were creeping in, getting closer to the petrol tank used for the starter motor. Then suddenly

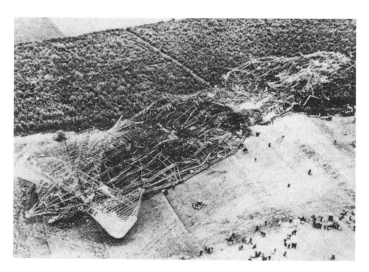

3.27 The remains of R 101, Bois de Coutumes, Beauvais, 5 October 1930.

a deluge of water came down – the fire had released some of the water ballast – and the flames around the car were extinguished. Binks and Ball were able to get out, pick their way across the field in pouring rain, and make contact with Leach and some of the other eight survivors (two of whom died later). Altogether 47 people were killed, including the Secretary of State for Air.

The fire could have been ignited by calcium flares that were suspended around the control car: it will be recalled that after the impact Harry Leach saw this car surrounded by flames. Hydrogen is commonly blamed for fire in the pre-war airships, but it has recently been suggested that the dope used for treating the cover might be a medium through which ignition would propagate at very high speed, such that the whole cover would burst into flames almost instantaneously. A catastrophic ignition of this sort is consistent with the reports of survivors.

The cause of the tragedy cannot be known with certainty. However, it is clear from survivors' evidence that the control car had been warned of a potential catastrophe. Joe Binks, as he came down from the crew quarters to the number 5 engine car, saw Michael Rope, assistant chief designer at the Royal Aircraft Works, making his way forward, apparently checking on the condition of the ship. It seems likely that Rope found a potentially fatal defect such as a major tear in the cover combined with deflation of the forward gasbags, and relayed this information to the control car by means of one of the speaking tubes that ran along the length of the ship. Consistent with this supposition is the known weakness of the cover in the nose sections, and the fact that the forward speed fell after the ship passed over Beauvais.

Faults and failures

This tragic and rather sorry story has been included here as an example of the potentially disastrous result of mixing politics and engineering. The Royal Aircraft Works was at one and the same time a contractor and the client: it was competing with a commercial organisation, Vickers, but at the same time was setting the rules. Not surprisingly, when it produced an inferior ship (as a glance at Table 3.4 will show) it disqualified the competitor and decided that its product was the only one suitable for the prestigious India route.

Subsequently, the whole programme was dictated by political considerations. The refit was scheduled to fit in with the date of a government conference. Because of this timing it was impossible to replace suspect parts of the cover, and in order to fit in with Lord Thomson's attendance at the conference, the tests required by the original specification were cancelled and even the substitute less onerous test was not properly completed.

Of course, even if all the engineering work and testing had been carried out satisfactorily, it is virtually certain that one or both of the airships would have come to grief within a few years. Most of the other big airships crashed, simply because they were only suitable for fair-weather operations, and by 1940 the few survivors had been grounded. Nevertheless the immediate fate of the R 101 and its distinguished passengers was the result of political pressure, which caused engineers not to complete work and tests which were essential for safety. And they were able to do this because, as a government agency, they could change the rules to suit political requirements.

The chemical industry

The Flixborough disaster

Marsh and McLennan[23] estimate the capital loss due to the explosion and fire in the caprolactam plant at Flixborough, England, as being US$167 million at 1997 prices, making it the fifth largest property loss of its type during the 30 years up to 1996. The human cost was relatively much higher; 28 were killed and 36 injured on the site, and outside the works perimeter 53 people were injured and 1821 houses together with 167 shops and factories were damaged to a greater or lesser degree. It was a very grievous accident.[24]

The Flixborough works

The plant was located on the east bank of the river Trent, close to where this river runs into the Humber estuary. It was near the village of Flixborough and three miles from the town of Scunthorpe in eastern England.

The site was originally used for the production of fertilisers, but in 1964 Nypro, jointly owned by Dutch State Mines and Fisons Ltd, bought it for the production of caprolactam, which is the raw material for the synthesis of Nylon 6. The caprolactam was at first produced via the hydrogenation of phenol to form cyclohexanone. Then in 1967 the company was restructured and the plant was expanded. At the same time the process was changed so that cyclohexanone was made by the oxidation of cyclohexane. The unit in which this operation was carried out was considered hazardous (only too correctly, in the event), since cyclohexane is a volatile liquid, boiling at about 80 °C, and any leakage could give rise to problems.

Nevertheless, it was located close to the control room and near to the laboratory and office block. None of these buildings had any protection against explosion and when the disaster occurred the control room was completely flattened, its occupants killed and all records destroyed. The accident took place just before 5 pm on Saturday, 1 June 1974, and the office block was unoccupied. Those in the laboratory managed to escape uninjured and were able to provide useful information about the place from which the vapour cloud originated.

The process

Figure 3.28 is a simplified process flow diagram of the cyclohexane oxidation unit. It includes a sketch of the bypass between reactors 4 and 6, and the 8 inch stainless steel line between the two separators S 2538 and S 2539. Both these items were considered as possible sources of the vapour leak.

The oxidation was carried out in a train of six reactors, which were stainless-clad carbon steel vessels set at successively lower levels so that flow between them was by gravity. The temperature was 155 °C and the pressure approximately 8.8 kg/cm^2. Pressure in the reactors was equalised by the offgas line and by keeping the connecting pipes half full of liquid.

Cyclohexane was oxidised by injecting air and catalyst into the reactors. About 6% of the cyclohexane was converted to cyclohexanone and cyclohexanol together with unwanted acidic by-products. The products passed to a series of mixers and separators where the acidic components were first neutralised by caustic soda solution. The products of this reaction were then separated into hydrocarbon and aqueous phases. The hydrocarbon was distilled to separate cyclohexanone and cyclohexanol, which were transferred to another unit for conversion to caprolactam. The residual cyclohexane was returned to the system via a steam-heated exchanger. Make-up was provided from a storage tank.

On start-up the system was first pressurised by nitrogen to 4 kg/cm^2, then the cyclohexane was heated to 155 °C, at which point the final pressure of 8.8 kg/cm^2 should have been reached owing to the vapour pressure of the liquid. During start-up, pressures sometimes went up to just over 9 kg/cm^2. The relief valves were set at 11 kg/cm^2.

Removal of reactor 5

On 27 March 1974 cyclohexane was found to be leaking from reactor 5 and the plant was shut down in order to investigate. The following morning it was found that a crack 6 ft long was visible on the outside of the reactor.

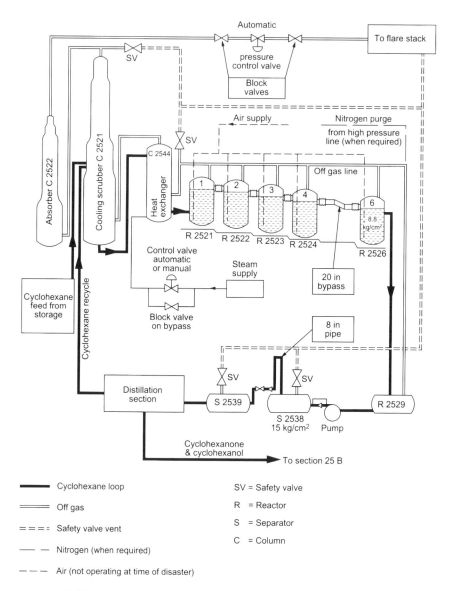

3.28 Simplified flow diagram of the cyclohexane plant at Flixborough.[23]

The vessels had been fabricated from $\frac{1}{2}$ in thick carbon steel clad with $\frac{1}{8}$ in stainless steel. The long crack was in the carbon steel backing material and as a result the stainless cladding was split over a shorter but unknown length. It was decided to remove the reactor for metallurgical examination and to construct a bypass to join reactors 4 and 6. This would enable production to continue.

It will be evident from Fig. 3.28 that the inlet nozzle for reactor 6 was lower than the outlet nozzle of reactor 4. To accommodate this difference a dog-leg-shaped pipe was fabricated with flanges that could be connected to the expansion bellows on the reactors. The original connecting pipes had a diameter of 28 in but the largest pipe available on site was 20 in, so this was used. The bypass was supported by scaffolding as shown in Fig. 3.29, with one cross-member under a flange and one under the pipe at each level. After the assembly had been bolted up and the scaffold support poles fixed as shown, a leak test was made with nitrogen at 4 kg/cm^2. A leak was found and repaired, the piping refitted, and a final pneumatic test was applied at 9 kg/cm^2. Construction codes for piping usually specify a hydraulic test at 1.3 times the design pressure, which at Nypro would have been just above the safety valve release pressure of 11 kg/cm^2. Such a pressure would have caused the bellows to fail and this would have precluded the catastrophe.

The reason for the fatal weakness, which of course was not realised by any of the Nypro staff at the time, is indicated in Fig. 3.30. Because of the displacement, the assembly as a whole is subject to forces which tend to make it rotate in a clockwise direction. At the same time there is a bending moment acting on the pipe which, if large enough, would cause it to buckle

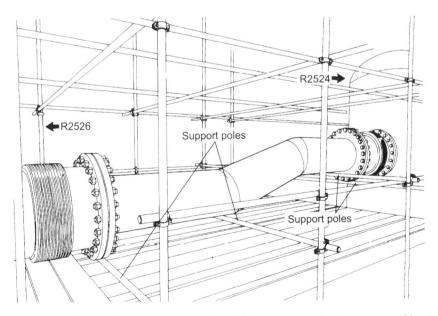

3.29 Probable arrangement of scaffolding supports for bypass assembly at Flixborough.[23]

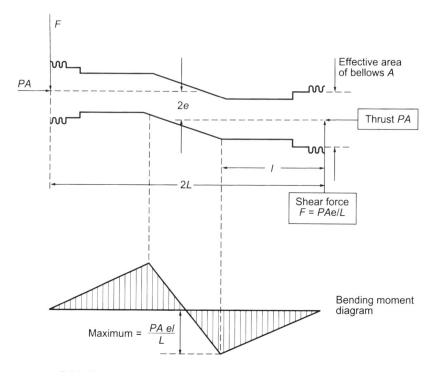

3.30 Shear forces and bonding moment on bypass assembly at Flixborough.[23]

at the mitre joints. The rotating force subjects the bellows to shear loads that they are not equipped to withstand. Bellows are made of relatively thin-walled material (in this instance austenitic stainless steel) and they can bend like a concertina, but if the bending goes too far the convolutions stretch out and the assembly is permanently damaged. Any further increase in pressure is then likely to result in a split or burst.

The works engineer 'a qualified mechanical engineer' had recently left the company and had not yet been replaced. No other person on site had the training or experience to understand these problems or to design piping systems. The 20-inch pipe was checked to ensure that it would withstand the temperature and pressure, otherwise the design work was limited to ensuring that the assembly was a good fit.

Operation with bypass in place

On 1 April start-up operations began and the plant ran normally for about two months. There were no problems with the bypass. There were two short shutdowns during this period but pressure was maintained throughout.

On 29 May a leak was discovered on the bottom isolating valve of a level indicator and the unit was shut down. The leak was repaired and on 1 June circulation of cyclohexane was started again. The start-up went somewhat irregular owing to further leaks and other problems. The last shift prior to the explosion was from 7 am to 3 pm on 1 June. It would appear that at the end of this shift the full operating temperature and pressure had still not been reached. The operators were required to circulate at the operating temperature and pressure for several hours before starting the air injection, so when the next shift took over at 3 pm normal operating conditions, including oxidation, were unlikely to be achieved for some time.

The explosion took place at 4.53 pm. It was a typical vapour cloud explosion caused by a massive release of cyclohexane. Experts estimated that the force generated was equivalent to the explosion of 15–45 tons of TNT. There was property damage over a wide area. Almost all the houses in the nearby village were damaged and the plant itself was largely destroyed.

The source of the vapour was undoubtedly the 28-inch openings in reactors 4 and 6 which had been formed when the bypass collapsed. The remains of this item were found on the plinth below the reactors. It had jack-knifed, bent through almost 180°. The other possible source of cyclohexane was a burst in the 8-inch stainless steel pipe joining the separators and shown diagrammatically in Fig. 3.28.

Tests on the bypass assembly

For reasons that were given earlier, the bypass was a most unsatisfactory arrangement and its collapse was almost certainly the immediate cause of the accident. However, since it had operated for two months without incident, it was considered necessary to determine its actual failure pressure.

To this end a similar piping rig was fabricated and was fitted between reactors 2 and 4, no. 3 having been removed. Scaffold supports were provided as in the original and the pipe was loaded internally with a chain to represent the weight of liquid. It was heated electrically to 155 °C and pressurised with nitrogen. The reactors were blanked off and filled with water. The results of the relevant tests are summarised in Table 3.5. Collapse of the bellows occurred at 9.8 kg/cm^2, only a little higher than the operating pressure, but they did not burst until the pressure was higher than the relief valve pressure. Other tests reinforced the result. The final conclusion was that under the experimental conditions, jack-knifing and bellows rupture would not occur at or near the normal operating conditions.

Table 3.5 Results of tests on simulated bypass assembly at Flixborough[23]

Scaffold support		Temperature (°C)	Test pressure (kg/cm²)	Result
No. of poles	Initial position			
5	In contact with pipe	155	8.8	No effect
5		155	8.8	No effect
4	Lowered ¼ inch (6 mm) to represent expansion of reactors	155	8.8	No effect
4		160	9.8	Bellows distorted
4		160	14.6	Bellows burst

The cause of the disaster

Examination of the 8-inch stainless steel line between the separators immediately after the accident showed, in addition to one large and one small rupture, numbers of fine cracks. At the time it seemed possible that these cracks were due to stress-corrosion cracking and that the failure had been a two-stage process; first a release of vapour from the 8-inch pipe, followed by an explosion causing the detachment of the bypass, followed in time by the main release of vapour and the explosion that destroyed the plant. However, examination of samples showed that the cracks were due to zinc embrittlement. If molten zinc is in contact with the surface of austenitic stainless steel at a temperature of 800 °C or more, intergranular cracking occurs. If this happens on the surface of a pipe under pressure, the pipe is likely to burst. At this point it should have been evident that the 8-inch pipe failure was the result of the fire, not the cause of it, particularly as there was no evidence of two successive explosions. Nevertheless, the experts advising Nypro persisted in supporting the two-stage rupture theory and much of the time of the inquiry was spent in examining, and then finally rejecting, this notion.

There remained the problem of explaining why the bypass failed at some pressure below 11 kg/cm², whereas in the tests a pressure of 14.6 kg/cm² was required for bursting. The test set-up was such that as the bellows convolutions blew out and the volume of the mock-up bypass increased, the pressure would tend to fall. Under operating conditions this would not happen; the pressure would remain steady and expansion of gas into the increased volume would result in a sudden input of energy. This would cause the other bellows to fail, which could generate sufficient energy for the pipe to jack-knife, tearing out the remains of the bellows and allowing large volumes of cyclohexane to vaporise. It was calculated that such an event would be likely to occur at a pressure between 10 kg/cm² and the relief valve setting of $11\,kg/cm^2$. Thus, a relatively modest increase in pressure could have triggered the failure.

The other possible cause would be an internal event leading to a sudden rise in pressure. Processes in which hydrocarbons are oxidised by air are notoriously subject to internal explosions. In the cyclohexane unit there was a known risk of explosion if the oxygen content of the off-gas line exceeded 5%, and detectors were in place against this contingency. However, oxidation had not started before the last shift took over, so this type of explosion is improbable. Other possibilities were explored by the court of inquiry but were likewise dismissed as improbable. Nevertheless, it must be recalled that the bypass performed satisfactorily, without visible distortion or other distress, for a period of two months before the explosion. During that time it must have been exposed to numerous pressure fluctuations, so that it had, as it were, been proof tested against normal operational variations. A sudden internal event would have provided a much more convincing explanation of the failure than the one described above, which was finally adopted by the court of inquiry. Unfortunately, the destruction of all the relevant records makes it impossible to explore this hypothesis other than in a speculative way.

The Flixborough disaster was the first major plant loss to be caused by a vapour cloud explosion following a full-bore rupture of piping. Such failures have subsequently resulted in a substantial proportion of vapour cloud explosions, which in turn have become a major cause of large hydrocarbon plant catastrophes. At the time the Flixborough failure was considered to be a direct result of incorrect design of the piping bypass, and this was in turn due to lack of engineering expertise on the site. This judgement needs to be modified in the light of later experience, which shows that large-scale vapour release can occur because of the rupture of piping that has been correctly designed in accordance with the relevant piping code.

Rail accidents

Collision involving the Los Angeles–Miami Express

In spite of the general fall in fatality rates due to rail accidents, major disasters continue to occur from time to time, often as a result of a combination of improbable circumstances. Such was the case with the accident which befell the Los Angeles–Miami Express in the early hours of 22 September 1993.[10]

Large quantities of bulk materials are imported through the port of Mobile, Alabama, which lies on the Gulf of Mexico. These materials are transported inland up the Mobile River by very large barges, which are pushed upstream by a tugboat. The *Mauvilla* was such a boat, and on the night in question was pushing six barges, three abreast and suitably fastened together. During the night a thick fog developed, and the pilot of the *Mauvilla* lost his way: instead of continuing up the Mobile River he turned up a subsidiary creek. At this time he was looking for an anchorage where he could tie up and wait for the fog to lift. The radar screen showed a barrier ahead. This the pilot interpreted as a moored tugboat with its barges spread across the river, and he decided to pull alongside and tie up. Shortly afterwards he felt a slight jolt and thought he had struck a sandbank. He extricated his craft and was subsequently occupied in rescuing surviving passengers from the river.

The following day investigators pieced together the sequence of events. The *Mauvilla* had collided, not with a sandbank, but with one of the concrete piers of the Big Bayou Canot railway bridge. Two of the forward barges were arrested by the impact, but the third broke loose and collided with the bridge itself, bending the rails into an S-shape. Meantime, the Los Angeles–Miami Express was approaching the bridge at 70 miles per hour. When the locomotive hit the kink in the track it shot up in the air, demolishing that part of the bridge which lay ahead, and then buried itself in the mud on the opposite bank of the creek. The front part of the train, consisting of double-decker coaches, ran straight into the water. Some passengers managed to escape and were either picked up by the *Mauvilla* or swam to the bridge and were eventually rescued by surviving members of the train crew.

The rear portion of the train remained either on the remains of the bridge or on dry land and the conductor was able to alert the emergency services by telephone. The pilot of the *Mauvilla* was at first quite unaware of the part he had played in this disaster, but in the end he did the right thing: he handed in his pilot's licence. There were 202 passengers on board the train at the time of the accident: 42 passengers and 5 crew members lost their lives, mostly by drowning.

The accident at Eschede

A very different type of railway accident occurred at Eschede, Germany on 3 June 1998.[25] Just after passing through Eschede station, the leading passenger car of a German Federal Railway high-speed train became derailed, as did the second and third vehicles. At the time, the train was passing under a concrete bridge. The first two coaches passed through, but the third slewed across the track, striking and demolishing two piers that supported the bridge, which started to collapse. The fourth and fifth vehicles went through with some damage, but the sixth was buried under the falling masonry. The seventh to twelfth cars then piled up on one another. One hundred persons were killed and 88 were injured in this accident.

The cause of the derailment was a broken tyre. There are two main types of railway wheel; the first is a monobloc, in which the wheel is machined from a solid casting. In the second type a forged steel ring (the tyre) is heated and then allowed to shrink on to a central disc, after which it is finish machined. The tyred wheel has the advantage that casting defects, if present, are not exposed on the rim. On the other hand, the shrink fit generates a residual tensile stress in the tyre, and this increases the severity of the fatigue loading cycle. Thus, if a crack-like defect is present in the forged ring, it could propagate and result in a catastrophic failure. This is probably what happened prior to the Eschede accident. Certainly such failures had occurred with similar tyred wheels on the Hamburg S-Bahn.

The German Federal Railway investigators produced their conclusions with commendable speed. The tyre, which was on one of the right-hand wheels, cracked about 6 km south of Eschede station. It ran on for slightly less than 300 m and then twisted upwards, lodging in the bogie. The train then continued for another 5.5 km in a stable fashion. South of Eschede station the rail layout includes a number of points. At Number 2 points the tyre was dislodged and hit a guard rail, which bent upwards and thrust into the interior of the first coach. The shock of the impact caused the left-hand wheel to come off the rail and strike Number 2 points, moving them in such a way that the coaches were derailed, with disastrous consequences.

It was, of course, almost inevitable that the train would be derailed when it hit the first sets of points after losing the tyre. The location, in this instance, was a most unlucky one. Other road bridges along the same line had been strengthened, and the supports set further back. Such was not the case at Eschede, and the collapse of the bridge contributed substantially to the severity of the accident.[26–28]

The opening of the Liverpool and Manchester Railway

The opening of the Liverpool and Manchester Railway took place on 15 September 1830. It should have been the celebration of an engineering triumph. Instead, it was a public relations and political disaster and for William Huskisson, who became the first passenger to be killed on a railway, a personal tragedy.

The Stockton to Darlington line, often quoted as the first passenger-carrying railway, had opened five years previously. It had, however, two features which would make such a claim questionable. In the first place, it was a common-user facility. This meant that it was open to horse-drawn as well as locomotive-drawn traffic. Although there were passing loops, this is not compatible with a regular service. Secondly, the passenger coaches were horse drawn; only coal trains were drawn by a locomotive. The Liverpool to Manchester line, on the other hand, was dedicated to locomotive-drawn trains, giving a scheduled service to passengers as well as carrying freight.

There had been doubts about the best means of haulage on the railway, whether by fixed engines or by locomotives. Fixed engines could haul loads up an incline, but if one engine broke down the whole railway could be halted. Accordingly the railway company decided to organise a competition for the best locomotive. The company set specifications, for example for maximum weight and steam pressure, and for the performance. The locomotive had to be capable of hauling a load of 20 tons at 10 mph regularly. Trials were to be conducted at Rainhill, where a level track was laid for the purpose. There was a prize of £500 for the winner. There were three contenders: of these Robert Stephenson's *Rocket* met both specifications and trials without difficulty, whilst the other two met neither. The company therefore ordered a number of similar engines from Robert Stephenson's works and these were built in good time for the opening.

The company had invited about 600 persons to take part in the ceremony. These included the Duke of Wellington, who was Prime Minister, Sir Robert Peel, a number of MPs including William Huskisson, MP for Liverpool, together with shareholders and leading citizens from Liverpool and Manchester. The most important persons were to be accommodated in one train and seven trains were provided for the remainder. The guests were to board their trains in Liverpool and proceed to the Manchester terminus, where lunch would be served. This was rather similar to the opening of the Stockton and Darlington line. Here there had been a remarkable display of public enthusiasm, with thousands of cheering spectators, while the celebratory dinner in Stockton Town Hall ended at midnight, after uncountable toasts had been drunk.

The Liverpool to Manchester Railway was a double track line, with crossings from one line to another at both termini and at Huyton, near Liverpool. For the opening, the Duke of Wellington's train was stationed on the south line and the others on the north. It was arranged that the Duke's special train should proceed to Parkside, a distance of a little under 20 miles, where the engine would pick up water, whilst the other trains steamed past. No doubt it was intended that the lesser guests should be seated at the lunch table by the time the great ones arrived. This operation was initiated successfully by firing a cannon and the trains were cheered on their way by a great multitude of Liverpool people.

Two of the trains on the north line had passed the stationary train at Parkside when some of the passengers on this train decided to alight in order to stretch their legs. The company had dumped sand on the permanent way and levelled it off flush with the top surface of the rails, with the object of aiding such perambulations. There were strict rules against disembarking between authorised stops, but no doubt it was felt that for such august persons and on such a day the normal rules did not apply. Nevertheless it was a most foolhardy act. At this point the railroad ran along the top of a dam or causeway, so that there was no escape to level ground on the far side of the track.

Huskisson had been President of the Board of Trade – a cabinet post – but had resigned some two years previously over an apparently trivial matter. Since then there had been a coolness between himself and the Prime Minister, a breach which colleagues were anxious to mend, and indeed this was accomplished, because as the company strolled along the track, the Duke, standing by the door of his carriage, held out his hand to Huskisson, who shook it warmly. At this point someone saw the third train, which was hauled by the *Rocket*, approaching and shouted a warning. All the perambulators were able either to scramble aboard or get into a safer position, except Huskisson who panicked, ran to and fro and eventually fell over with one leg across the line. The *Rocket* had no brakes and could only be stopped in an emergency by putting the engine in reverse, an operation requiring great skill. This manoeuvre was accomplished, but not before Huskisson had been run over and grievously hurt. The flesh and bones of the thigh were crushed and the artery severed. He was at once attended by two Liverpool doctors, who stopped the arterial bleeding by means of a tourniquet.

George Stephenson had meantime caused the leading coach of the special train, which on the outward journey had housed a military band, to be uncoupled. Huskisson was lifted on to an improvised stretcher (a door) and put on board this carriage, accompanied by Lord Wilton and others. Stephenson then drove to Eccles, where the injured man was taken to the vicarage. The vicar, the Rev. Thomas Blackburne, was a friend of Huskisson. More doctors were called but they could do no more than provide laudanum to deaden the pain. Between 9 and 10 that evening, Huskisson died.

Amongst those left behind there was a long debate about procedure. The Duke and Sir Robert Peel were in favour of returning to Liverpool, but were eventually persuaded to continue by the Borough Reeve of Manchester, who argued that the large crowd waiting in the Manchester terminus might riot if the trains did not arrive.

This was speculation and very wide of the mark. Manchester was the heartland of agitation for parliamentary reform, where the Duke of

Wellington was regarded as the chief enemy of the cause. So an anti-government demonstration had been set up and in spite of calling out the army, the mob had invaded the Manchester terminus.

Meanwhile, the Duke's train, being without an engine, was lashed to a train on the north track and dragged in this way to Eccles, where Stephenson was stationed with *Northumbrian* (Fig. 3.31). This was connected up and the trains were able to proceed in good order.

Some of the demonstrators had by now reached the cutting ahead of Manchester station so when the trains arrived here they were met by a hostile crowd waving banners and throwing stones and brickbats. The engines were slowed down to a crawl and there were no casualties. Eventually all arrived at Manchester station. Here the situation was confusing. Most of the waiting crowd was antagonistic, largely due to ill feeling towards the government and towards the Duke of Wellington in particular. But there also seemed to be some hostility towards the railway itself, in line with a suspicion of new machinery, which had been prevalent in England for many years. At the same time there were numbers of enthusiastic supporters and others who were just curious.

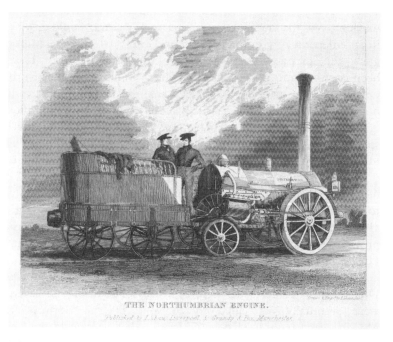

THE NORTHUMBRIAN ENGINE.

3.31 The steam locomotive *Northumbrian*, which was driven by George Stephenson at the opening of the Liverpool to Manchester Railway (courtesy of Science & Society Picture Library).

By about 3pm, some of the guests were bold enough or hungry enough to struggle across to the area where lunch was to be provided, but most remained in their seats. The Duke likewise remained in his carriage and eventually the Manchester police chief got through to recommend a return to Liverpool. The order for a retreat was given and the special train started on the return trip. Unfortunately four of the engines from the other trains had already set off on the same track to Eccles in order to pick up water. These engines would need to return nearly to Liverpool in order to cross over to the other line, so only three engines remained for the seven trains. It took a long time to detach these engines and for them to proceed to Eccles for water and to return. Darkness had then fallen and it had started to rain.

The engineers decided that it would be best to couple all the carriages together to form one long train and to haul this with the three engines. After some manoeuvring this was achieved and the new long train got under way. There was a stop at Eccles to enquire about Huskisson. On attempting to restart, two couplings broke. The carriages were lashed together with ropes and the train restarted. At Parkside three of the missing engines appeared, one having gone ahead of the special train as pilot, looking for obstacles. Two of the three were coupled to the head of the train, and one sent ahead, again as a pilot. The only lighting available at this time was by burning lengths of tallow rope, so the pilot was a sensible precaution.

It was 10pm by the time that the train reached Liverpool, but on this occasion the waiting crowd cheered and welcomed the sorely tried passengers. The journey ended with a descent by cable through a sloping tunnel to Wapping Dock and the guests finally departed at 11pm. Late, but it must be remembered that in a day marked by human disaster and malevolence, there had only been one mechanical failure: the entirely excusable breakage of the couplings at Eccles. Otherwise the engines and rolling stock had performed impeccably.

The following morning the first scheduled service left Liverpool for Manchester with 140 passengers on board. The railway age had begun. But it was 13 years before the Duke of Wellington made another journey by train.

Comment

There are some disasters from which there is no escape. When a passenger aircraft falls out of the sky it is a near certainty that all therein will be killed. Most catastrophes, however, are more tolerant. In the case of floods, for example, timely evacuation of those who are threatened can greatly reduce the loss of life. In maritime disasters there is often a possibility of rescue, particularly in recent years. The final outcome, though, may be much affected by human behaviour, as shown in some of the cases described earlier in this chapter.

The loss of the *Sea Gem* provides a characteristic example. After the platform had fallen into the sea from a height of about 60 feet, the drillers and some others prepared to evacuate by inflatable rafts. Other members of the crew had climbed up to or near the heli deck. When called upon to board the life rafts, these men did not respond and, in spite of heroic efforts by the others, they had to be left on board, to drown when the rig sank shortly afterwards.

On the *Alexander L Kielland*, whilst some managed to board lifeboats and others swam towards a neighbouring platform, others climbed to the highest point on the wreck and stayed there until it capsized. Most of those who mustered on the upper deck of *Piper Alpha* stayed there and died, whilst most of those who jumped into the sea were saved. Many of the passengers who were left on board the *Titanic* gathered together on the stern as the ship began to sink.

It would seem that the bold, who take to the sea after a disaster, have a good chance of being saved, whilst the less bold, who cling to the wreckage, do not.

Communication

It is often said that failures of communication are a potent cause of accident in human activities. The loss of the *Titanic* is sometimes cited as a case in point, and of course this may be justified on the grounds that if the officers of the *Californian* had identified the rockets they saw as disaster signals, and if they had roused the radio operator, then they would have known about the collision with the iceberg and could have steamed to the rescue. Whether the *Californian* would have arrived in time is another matter.

In fact the history of that night is rather one of the failure of human perception. First, of course, was the failure to spot the iceberg. However explicable or excusable, this was nevertheless a failure. Secondly, passengers and crew on the sinking ship saw the masthead lights of a steamer, and this steamer appeared to be coming towards them. It was this observation that caused Boxhall, quartermaster of the watch on the *Titanic*, to fire distress rockets. But the steamer never appeared nor was it identified subsequently.

On the *Californian* a vessel, thought to be a small or medium-sized tramp steamer, was seen around midnight at a distance of about 5 miles. The captain was concerned to keep his distance so the ship was kept under observation. The second officer of the *Californian*, Mr Stone, saw the rocket flashes and assumed that they came from this second vessel but they did not appear to be distress rockets and eventually the ship steamed off. Again, this vessel was never identified.

The picture is a confused one. The best interpretation seems to be that the *Californian* and the *Titanic* were not in sight of each other. The flashes seen from the *Californian* were in fact Boxhall's rockets. Their explosions were not heard on the *Californian* either because of distance or as a result of some freak atmospheric condition.

The *Piper Alpha* disaster has also been categorised as being due to a failure of communication. The day-shift operators did not, it is thought, tell the night shift that a safety valve had been removed from one of the compressors, and the paperwork gave no indication of this fact. Consequently it was possible, simply by signing a piece of paper, for one of the night-shift operators to pressurise a compressor that was in an unsafe condition. In addition to the failure to communicate between individuals, the control system was evidently inadequate. There is much merit in the physical identification of out-of-service equipment on the piece of equipment itself (flagging) as specified by the Minerals Management Service of the US Department of the Interior. It is proposed to extend this system to control panels, pumps and flow control valves upstream of such equipment. A direct means of communication, such as flagging, is more likely to be effective than an indirect system.

Human error figures largely as a cause of failure in the record of aircraft accidents. In many cases, however, some deficiency in the control system may play an important part. The Comet that broke up in a storm after taking off from Calcutta airport was a case in point: the rudder control had no 'feel' so that the pilot may have inadvertently applied excessive force to it, resulting in a structural failure. Another example was the loss of an aircraft at Stockton, UK, in 1967. This crash was caused by engine failure, which in turn was due to leaving a valve in a crossfeed fuel line partly open. This valve was controlled by a lever, where the correct position was indicated by a detent, or spring-loaded notch. The detent had become worn and once again the 'feel' of the control was lost. On the other hand, in an aircraft crash that occurred in 1989, one of the engines of a twin-engined jet started to fail. The crew intended to shut down the defective engine but instead, by a serious error of judgement, shut down the good engine. This was indubitably a case of human error.

Fatigue cracking

The two Comet aircraft losses in the Mediterranean were entirely due to errors in design and in no way to pilot error. In this, and in other respects, the character of this failure was remarkably similar to that which led to the loss of the *Alexander L Kielland* 26 years later. Both were due to unstable fast fractures initiated by a fatigue crack, and in both cases the fatigue crack was initiated by a point of stress concentration at the edge of a circular opening. In the case of the *Alexander L Kielland* the partial failure of a piece of plate under transverse loading, which caused disbonding and lack of reinforcement around the opening, made a major contribution to the failure. Other similar design features, where there was no disbonding, had behaved satisfactorily at least up to the time of the disaster. The metal used to construct the Comet was not in any way defective. However, it does seem likely that a failure of the adhesive bonding between the aircraft skin and the window reinforcement may have occurred at some stage: in at least one of the post-crash tests the skin rode over a rivet head.

In neither case was any fatigue analysis carried out in the initial stages of design, it being thought that a safety factor used in establishing the design stress would avoid fatigue problems. In neither case was there any redundancy in the design, so that the initial failure caused a catastrophic disruption of the structure as a whole. In both cases the designers were venturing into a new field where previous experience was very limited.

It would be unreasonable to suggest that if the Pentagone designers (or Lloyd's Register, which also participated) had studied the Comet failures, the *Alexander L Kielland* tragedy would have been averted. Nevertheless, a study of both these failures would be of benefit to all engineers who might be concerned with the design of structures subject to fatigue loading. Even where there is previous experience with a particular type of structure, it must be remembered that apparently minor changes in design can result in the initiation of a fatigue crack.

Vapour cloud explosions

Two of the catastrophes discussed in the chapter were due to vapour cloud explosions. The *Piper Alpha* and the Flixborough disasters underline one common feature: namely, the handling of potentially explosive substances. Gaseous hydrocarbons and hydrogen fall into this category as a matter of course. Cyclohexane would normally be regarded as a volatile and inflammable liquid, in the same category as gasoline. However, at high temperature and pressure the hazard of handling this substance is of a different order; the explosion risk is, if anything, greater than with gaseous hydrocarbons because of the large mass of vapour that can be generated by the failure of equipment, as demonstrated at Flixborough. Gas leak detectors and dispersion systems offer no defence against a full-bore rupture in plant handling such substances because – as on *Piper Alpha* –

by the time the operator has noted the alarm, or very shortly afterwards, the vapour cloud will have exploded.

The causes of major leaks in process plant are very diverse. Accidents may result from faults in design, in construction, in operation or maintenance, or they may be due to natural hazards. Analysts concerned with risk reduction must, therefore, cover a wide range of possible events.

References

1. 'And yet the band played on', *The Times*, 26 May 1994.
2. Garzke, W.H., Yoerger, D.R., Harris, S., Dulin, R.O. and Brown, D.K. 'Deep underwater exploration vehicles – past, present and future', paper presented at the Centennial meeting of the Society of Naval Architects and Marine Engineers, New York City, 1992.
3. Ballard, R.D. *The Discovery of the 'Titanic'*, Madison Press Books, Toronto, 1987.
4. Bone, James, 'How fragile steel condemned the "Titanic" on freezing seas', *The Times*, 17 September 1993.
5. Spouge, J.R. 'The safety of Ro-Ro passenger ferries', *Trans RINA* 1989 **131** 1–12.
6. Spouge, J.R. 'Passenger ferry safety in the Philippines', *Trans RINA* 1990 **132** 179–88.
7. Hooke, N. *Modern Shipping Disasters 1963–1987*, Lloyd's of London Press, London, 1989.
8. Harris, J. 'Boredom and the human factor in accidents', *Mater. World* 1994 **2** 590.
9. Jubb, J. *Structural Failure of Bulk Carriers*, Thomas Lowe Gray lecture 1995. Institution of Mechanical Engineers, London.
10. Faith, N. *Mayday*, Channel 4 Books, Macmillan, London, 1998.
11. Anon, 'The *Alexander L Kielland* accident', *Norwegian Public Reports* Nov. 1981 **11** (English translation).
12. Gurney, T.R. *Fatigue of Welded Structures*, Cambridge University Press, London, 1968.
13. Gurney, T.R. 'Fatigue design rules for welded steel joints', *Welding Institute Res. Bull.* 1976 **17** 115.
14. Cullen, W.D. 'The public inquiry into the *Piper Alpha* disaster', Cm 1310, Her Majesty's Stationery Office, London, 1990.
15. Danenberger, E.P. and Schneider, R.R. '*Piper Alpha* – the US regulatory response', in *Offshore Operations Post Piper Alpha*, Institute of Marine Engineers and RINA, London, 1991.
16. *Offshore Operations Post Piper Alpha*, Institute of Marine Engineers and RINA, London, 1991, p. 193.
17. Anon, 'Piper B platform is installed in North Sea', *Marine Eng. Rev.* 1991, 64.
18. Kennedy, J., Linzi, P. and Dennis, P. 'The safety background to the design of the Tiffany platform', in *Offshore Operations Post Piper Alpha*, Institute of Marine Engineers and RINA, London, 1991, pp. 81–90.

19. Report of the court of inquiry into the accidents to Comet G-ALYP on 10th January 1954 and Comet G-ALYY on 8th April 1954, Her Majesty's Stationery Office, London, 1955.
20. Wells, A.A. *The Conditions for Fast Fracture in Aluminium Alloys with Particular Reference to the Comet Failures*, BWRA Research Report RB 129, April 1955.
21. Shute, N. *Slide Rule*, Heinemann, London, 1972.
22. Masefield, P.G. *To Ride the Storm*, William Kimber, London, 1982.
23. Mahoney, D. *Large Property Damage Losses in the Hydrocarbon-chemical Industries – a Thirty-year Review*, Marsh and McLennan, Chicago, 1997.
24. Anon, *The Flixborough Disaster*, Her Majesty's Stationery Office, London, 1975.
25. Gough, J. and Kemnitz, J. 'Eschede: the aftermath', *Modern Railways*, August 1988 524–5.
26. Rolt, L.T.C. *George and Robert Stephenson*, Longman, London, 1971.
27. Ferneyhough, F. *Liverpool and Manchester Railway 1830 to 1980*, Robert Hale, London, 1980.
28. Fay, C.R. *Huskisson and his Age*, Longmans Green, 1951.

CHAPTER 4

The technical background

The record has shown that a significant proportion of catastrophic failures are initiated by the unexpected fracture of some part of the structure; the capsizing of the *Alexander L. Kielland* rig and the explosive rupture of the Comet aircraft being two examples described in the previous chapter. Mechanical failure is also the most frequent cause of loss in the hydrocarbon processing industry.

The other problem that is an increasing scourge in hydrocarbon processing, and which continues to affect shipping and offshore operations, is explosions, particularly of hydrocarbon–air mixtures. The character of explosions and the ways in which they initiate and propagate are discussed later in this chapter.

Mechanical failure

The type of mechanical failure that, with good reason, occasions most concern is that which takes place under normal operating conditions. The fracture mode which, in the past, gave rise to such failures was low-stress brittle fracture, whilst fatigue cracking remains a serious problem. Under this heading it is proposed, therefore, to review first the mechanisms of brittle fracture and the various ways in which metals, and steel in particular, may be embrittled. Then some cases where structures have suffered undesirable modes of fast fracture when severely loaded will be described. Finally, the mechanical failures giving rise to the catastrophic failure of process plant are considered.

The fracture of brittle solids

If a uniform tensile stress σ is applied to a plate of a brittle material, say glass, it will be strained elastically by an amount σ/E, where E is the elastic modulus. In this process, work is done and such work is stored in the plate as strain energy. If the amount of strain is ε then the strain energy content of the plate is $\frac{1}{2}\sigma\varepsilon$ per unit volume. This may also be expressed as $\frac{1}{2}\sigma^2/E$, and the relevant SI units are, for example, joules per cubic metre. If a small crack of length $2a$ is introduced into such a plate, the strain energy around the crack will be reduced by an amount equal to $\pi\sigma^2a^2/E$. This result, which at the time had recently been obtained by Inglis, was used by Griffith[1] in a paper published in 1920 to develop a theory of brittle fracture. The crack makes two contributions to the energy of the system: a negative one, due to the reduction of strain energy, and a positive one, due to the formation of two new surfaces. If the sum of these quantities increases with increasing crack length, the system is stable, but if the contrary is true, then the crack will extend in a catastrophic manner. More generally crack extension occurs when the value of σ^2a rises to a critical level. This rule was used in the previous chapter in connection with the explosive failures of Comet aircraft.

The rate at which strain energy is lost as the crack length increases is $\mathrm{d}/\mathrm{d}a\left(\dfrac{\pi^2a^2}{E}\right)=\dfrac{2\pi^2a}{E}$. At the point of instability this quantity is equal to the rate at which energy is absorbed by the formation of new surfaces. Beyond this point, however, the rate of energy release is predicted to continue increasing indefinitely. It would be expected, therefore, that the crack velocity should increase sharply until other forces come into play.

Crack velocity in glass has been the subject of many studies, mainly at the University of Freiburg, Germany and the Research Institute at Saint-Louis, France. This work has been summarised by Schardin.[2]

Most of the research was carried out using a multiple-spark high-speed camera, capable of 10^5 to 10^6 frames per second. A plate specimen was held in tension between fixed grips. A fracture was initiated by impact, and the camera was activated simultaneously. The progress of the crack tip (or tips, when the crack branched) could then be plotted as a function of time.

Figure 4.1 gives an example of such a plot. Initially a rapid increase in velocity is indicated but for the main part of the crack the velocity is constant. This constant velocity is independent of the stress applied to the sample and varies only slightly with temperature. It does, however, vary with the type of glass. There is quite a wide variation of physical and mechanical properties depending on the chemical composition of the glass. It is clearly of interest to explore possible correlations between fracture velocity and glass properties.

It is natural, in this connection, to look at a possible relationship between crack velocity and that of elastic waves. Some workers in this field have proposed that the fracture velocity should be one-half the velocity of shear (transverse) waves, but Schardin[2] has pointed out that the ratio between these two quantities varies with the type of glass. Moreover, the tests were conducted under tension, not shear. Accordingly, in Fig. 4.2 fracture velocities are plotted as a function of compression wave velocity, as

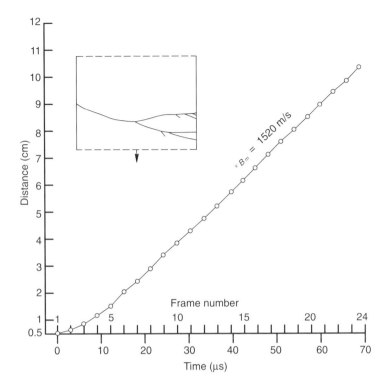

4.1 Displacement of the crack tip for a glass plate held at a constant stress of 8.8 MN/m². Inset sketch shows the form of the crack.

calculated from $(E/\rho)^{1/2}$. In this expression E is the elastic modulus in tension and ρ is density: where comparisons have been made, such values agree well with those obtained experimentally.

The correlation is good, the correlation coefficient for the regression line being 0.8734. This is a purely empirical observation; there is no generally accepted theory for crack propagation. It seems possible that elastic waves caused by the fracture generate stresses high enough to maintain crack growth and to override any pre-existing stress field.

Also included in the diagram is a plot for steel; this represents fracture velocities of 963–1090 m/s, as given by Schardin.[2] Robertson,[3] using a less sophisticated technique than those reported by Schardin, and under severe impact conditions, measured fracture velocities of 4000–6000 ft/s (1219–1829 m/s) in mild-steel plate. In this instance the fracture velocity was found to increase with the level of applied stress. A similar observation was made in the case of fractures in plexiglass. Plexiglass is a transparent

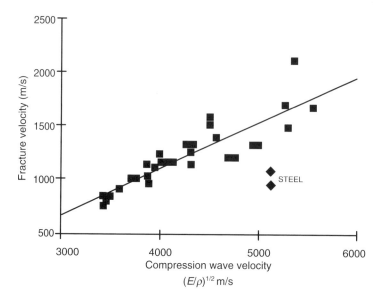

4.2 Fracture velocity of different types of glass as a function of compression wave velocity, calculated from $(E/\rho)^{1/2}$.[2]

polymer that has a degree of plasticity. In tests conducted in a manner similar to those for glass, it was found that the velocity built up to a constant maximum value, but this value increased with the amount of preapplied stress.

It was observed by Robertson that the rate of relaxation of strain after fracture of an elastic body must be finite. Such an effect might limit the rate of strain energy release, and thereby the velocity, of a fast-running crack.[4]

Fracture mechanics

In the years immediately following the Second World War, brittle failures of wartime shipping caused renewed interest in the work of Griffith, notably at the Naval Research Laboratory in Washington, DC. However, the main line of development was based on a technique for calculating the stress field around the tip of the crack. The result takes the form of an infinite series in successive half-powers of (ra): $-\frac{1}{2}$, 0, $\frac{1}{2}$, $\frac{3}{2}$ etc, r being the distance from the crack tip and a the crack length. It is assumed that r/a is small, so that the first term of the series is dominant. This is a linear approximation, the discipline first being called 'linear elastic fracture mechanics'. Having made this approximation, the stress field is proportional to a stress intensity factor, K, which in turn is equal to $k\sigma a^{1/2}$, where k is a constant, σ is stress and a the crack length. The stress intensity factor has a suffix I, II or III, according to whether the cracking is due to tension, shear or torsion, and a further suffix C for the value at which the crack starts to propagate. Thus, K_{IC} is the critical value for the initiation of fracture in tension (also known as the 'opening mode').

It will be recalled that the Griffith criterion for crack extension is that the rate of strain energy release should be equal to or exceed the rate of absorption of energy due to the formation of new surfaces, which for a brittle substance is 2γ, being the surface energy. This leads to the condition $(\sigma^2 a)_C$ = constant, so clearly the rate of release of strain energy, which is designated G, is related to the stress intensity factor. Specifically, we have $G = (1 - v^2) K^2/E$, where v is the Poisson ratio. The suffixes used for G are the same as for K, so that $G_{IC} = (1 - v^2) K_{IC}^2/E$.

The quantity G is clearly a material property, and its SI units are Joules per square metre (J/m^2). On the other hand, K_{IC} is a factor that is proportional to the intensity of the stress field immediately adjacent to the crack tip at the point of fracture. It is not a material property, but is widely quoted as such and is called 'fracture toughness'.

The fracture toughness of materials

Fracture toughness may be measured using the type of testpiece illustrated in Fig. 4.3. This specimen contains a machined edge crack which is extended by fatigue loading to give a sharp-tipped crack of total length a. It is loaded in tension using pins which pass through the indicated holes. A formula then relates K_{IC} to the load at failure. The result obtained is regarded as valid provided that the specimen thickness B exceeds $2.5 (K_{IC}/\sigma_y)^2$, where σ_y is yield strength. This condition is readily met in the case of brittle materials and high tensile steel, but for mild steel in a notch-ductile condition the required testpiece would be impracticably thick. However, it is found empirically that there is a relationship between the fracture toughness of unembrittled steel tested at room temperature and its yield strength:

$$K_{IC} = 225 - 0.1\sigma_y \qquad\qquad [4.1]$$

where K_{IC} is in $MN/m^{3/2}$ and σ_y is in MN/m^2. This formula indicates that the fracture toughness of mild steel in a good notch-ductile condition would be about $200\,MN/m^{3/2}$. This figure is included in Table 4.1, which gives the fracture toughness of various metallic and non-metallic materials.

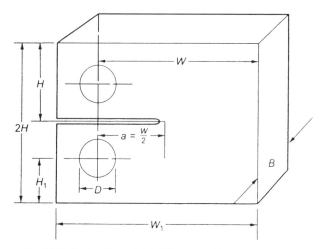

$W = 2.0B$, $D = 0.5B$, $a = 1.0B$, $W_1 = 2.5B$, $H = 1.2B$, $H_1 = 0.65B$

4.3 ASTM compact tension testpiece for the measurement of fracture toughness.

Table 4.1 Fracture toughness properties

Substance	Fracture toughness K_{IC} (MN/m$^{3/2}$)
Age-hardened aluminium alloy	50
Alumina	3–5
Brick	1–2
Carbon fibre reinforced plastic	60
Concrete	0.3
Epoxy resin	0.6–1.0
Glass fibre reinforced plastic	90
Glass (soda)	0.7
Ice	0.1
Steel, high tensile	65
Steel, medium tensile	180
Steel, mild	200
Zirconia	12

The fracture toughness of steel

Fracture toughness is a major factor in determining the reliability of engineering structures. In the case of non-heat-treatable aluminium alloys, which may be used for ship superstructures, fast unstable fracture has never been a problem, whilst the catastrophic failure of age-hardened alloys, such as caused the Comet I aircraft disasters, has not occurred subsequently. It is, therefore, the fracture toughness of steel with which we are mainly concerned.

Steel may suffer a loss of fracture toughness in a number of ways. In common with other metals that have a body-centred cubic crystal lattice structure, iron and steel have a transition temperature above which they behave in a relatively ductile manner and below which they are, in the presence of a notch, relatively brittle. Steel may undergo embrittling metallurgical changes, mainly due to service at elevated temperature or exposure to radioactive processes. Steel may crack due to the presence of dissolved hydrogen, either during fabrication using a fusion welding process, or in hydrogen service. These various modes of embrittlement are described below.

The effect of temperature

The ductile/brittle transition temperature for any given sample of steel is traditionally measured by breaking a notched bar in a pendulum-type impact tester and measuring the energy absorbed in the fracture. Tests are carried out over a range of temperatures and ideally the plot of absorbed energy against temperature gives an S-shaped curve. Figure 4.4 shows such

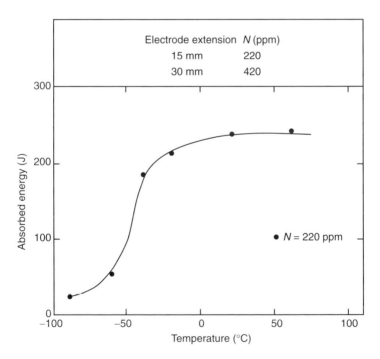

4.4 Charpy V-notch curve for a 0.06C 0.5Ni steel weld metal (after Boniszewski[5]).

a transition curve. There is a more or less horizontal lower portion (the lower shelf) joined by a steep line to a more or less horizontal upper portion (the upper shelf). The transition temperature range is defined by the vertical line, −50 °C to −40 °C in this case. Very often, however, the transition occurs over a much wider temperature range. It is therefore general practice to define the transition temperature as that where the absorbed energy reaches some minimum value, 27 J being a figure commonly accepted in European countries.

At temperatures below the transition, steel plates containing a sharp crack may fail in a brittle fashion if the crack is long enough and the applied stress high enough. However, as noted in the case of the *Titanic*, uncracked material will behave in a normally ductile fashion if stressed or bent at such temperatures. Figure 4.5 shows the properties of a medium-tensile steel (ASTM A 533) that has been used in the fabrication of thick-walled pressure vessels for nuclear power plant. These are plotted as a function of temperature for the range −300 °F to +100 °F (−184 °C to +38 °C). The upper diagram shows the fracture toughness transition curve as determined by the standard ASTM test. Also indicated are the nil ductility temperature (labelled NDT at 0 °F) and the 50% brittle fracture appearance Charpy impact transition temperature (labelled T_{50}, at about 80 °F). There is no standard minimum acceptance level for K_{IC}; the fracture toughness test is too costly for quality control purposes and it is not applicable to normal structural grades of steel. But the material was undoubtedly of good notch-ductile quality at room temperature.

The lower diagram shows the ductility as measured in a normal tensile test. There is hardly any change in elongation or reduction of area over the transition temperature range, and values only start to fall below about −200 °F. In other words, steel may behave in a brittle manner at low atmospheric temperatures but such behaviour is exceptional and requires either impact loading or the presence of a sharp crack, or a combination of these conditions. This conclusion is consistent with the behaviour of steel structures in general service.

The risk of brittle failure is, self-evidently, reduced by lowering the ductile–brittle transition temperature to a level below that at which the structure is required to operate. For low-carbon (mild) steel in the unembrittled condition, the most important factor in this respect is the grain size. The finer the grain, the lower is the transition temperature. Grain size, in turn, is determined by the rolling schedule to which the steel is exposed in forming plates or sections. The means of controlling such schedules to obtain optimum properties are described in Chapter 5.

Process plant may be required to operate at temperatures well below 0 °C. The addition of nickel to steel lowers the transition temperature,

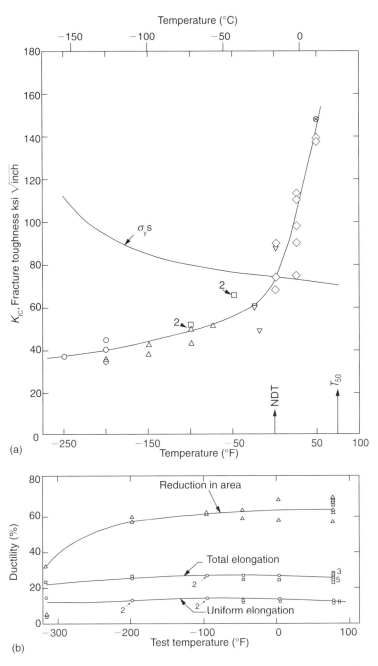

4.5 Properties of a medium-tensile pressure vessel steel as a function of temperature: (a) fracture toughness and yield strength; (b) ductility as measured in a normal tensile test (after Wessel[6]).

Table 4.2 Material selection for cold service: ASME Boiler and Pressure Vessel Code section VIII

Material	Temperature range	
	°F	°C
Austenitic chromium–nickel steel:		−196 to −101
9% nickel steel	−320 to −151	
3½% nickel steel	−150 to −51	−100 to −46
Impact tested carbon steel:		
normalised steel	−50 to −21	−45 to −29
fine-grained steel	−20 to −10	−28 to 21

whilst the austenitic chromium–nickel steels have a face-centred cubic lattice structure and may be used safely down to very low temperatures. Table 4.2 shows the permissible temperature range for various materials according to the ASME Boiler and Pressure Vessel Code. This schedule is widely used for process plant fabrication in the case of both pressure vessels and piping. Carbon steel with controlled impact properties is used for temperatures down to −50 °F.

Embrittlement mechanisms

Two modes of embrittlement have been associated with brittle fracture in steel: strain ageing and temper embrittlement.

Strain ageing occurs when steel containing free (uncombined) nitrogen is strained and heated, either simultaneously or at a later time, to a temperature in the region of 200 °C. Embrittlement results from the incipient precipitation of nitrides.

During the 1930s a number of welded steel bridges were erected in Belgium and Germany. These were fabricated from Bessemer converter steel which, because of the nature of the process, may contain free nitrogen. Several of these bridges failed by brittle fracture and it was found that small cracks caused by welding had suffered strain-ageing at the tip. Such embrittled short cracks are very effective in the initiation of unstable fracture. The remedy was to add small amounts of aluminium to the steel. This removes the free nitrogen and at the same time refines the grain and increases the yield strength. Only a relatively small amount of Bessemer steel is now produced, so the problem is unlikely to recur.

Temper embrittlement is an old problem. It was first observed by blacksmiths during the nineteenth century. Horseshoes that were tempered and then cooled in air could be brittle (hence the name) and it was found necessary to quench them in water.

When steel is heated to a high temperature it transforms to a face-centred cubic phase known as austenite. On cooling it reverts to the body-centred cubic form, ferrite, but the original austenite grain boundaries remain. These are regions where the lattice structure is disoriented and impurity atoms tend to diffuse thereto. Such diffusion takes place on slow cooling from a little below 600 °C and may cause embrittlement. The degree of embrittlement depends on the alloy composition, on the concentration of impurities and on the cooling rate.

The earliest American oil wells yielded a low-sulphur crude oil that could be distilled in unalloyed steel tubes. Later discoveries, however, corroded mild steel at an unacceptable rate, and 5% chromium tubes were employed to counter this problem. After a period of service this alloy became almost as brittle as glass owing to temper embrittlement, in this instance, due to holding at elevated temperature rather than slow cooling. The addition of small amounts of molybdenum prevented such embrittlement and gave rise to a family of chromium–molybdenum alloys which proved to have good mechanical properties at elevated temperatures as well as good resistance to sulphur corrosion.

One such alloy contains $2\frac{1}{4}$% chromium and 1% molybdenum. This has found a wide application for heavy-wall pressure vessels such as hydrocracker reactors. Unfortunately molybdenum does not offer complete protection against temper embrittlement and there was at least one case where such a vessel suffered a brittle fracture during repair operations. Several boiler drums failed in a brittle manner during hydrostatic testing in the 1960s. In these cases the embrittling agent was copper, an intentionally added alloying element. The alloy concerned is no longer in use.

It appears likely that the reduction of impact strength resulting from the post-weld heat treatment of pressure vessels is due to temper embrittlement. Improvements in the purity of steel should help to minimise this and other similar problems.

Embrittlement and cracking due to hydrogen

Hydrogen dissolves readily in steel at high temperature, for example, in the liquid weld pool during fusion welding. At room temperature or thereabouts it will only dissolve if the gas is very low in oxygen content (generally less than ten parts per million oxygen). Alternatively, it will dissolve at room temperature if it is in atomic form. This may happen during corrosion, when hydrogen is liberated in the presence of hydrogen sulphide, which has the effect of preventing hydrogen atoms from combining to form H_2 molecules.

Dissolved hydrogen has little effect on the properties of steel except within the temperature range −100 to 200 °C. Within this range the gas segregates to discontinuities: in particular to grain boundaries, to metal/inclusion interfaces and to parts that have been plastically strained, such as the tip of a crack. Where hydrogen concentrates in this way the cohesion of the metal lattice is reduced, and if the region is subject to tensile stress, a crack may form and propagate. Because it acts in this way, hydrogen reduces the fracture toughness of steel and it is possible to measure this reduced quantity, which is designated K_H. The value of K_H as a function of yield strength is plotted for quenched and tempered steels in Fig. 4.6. Hydrogen cracking is a time-dependent process: a true minimum value of K_H is obtained when the rate of strain, and the corresponding crack growth rate, are low enough to allow hydrogen to diffuse into and saturate the plastic zone at the crack tip. Few investigators have observed this requirement and therefore the data points scatter widely upwards.

Hydrogen cracking is a familiar characteristic of fusion welds made with damp coated electrodes or too low a preheat. The cracking usually occurs in the most susceptible parts, i.e. those having the highest yield strength or hardness. In carbon steel this is usually the weld metal, but in alloy steel it is commonly the heat-affected zone. When the stress intensity is low, the cracking is intergranular, but when high it is transgranular. The rate of crack

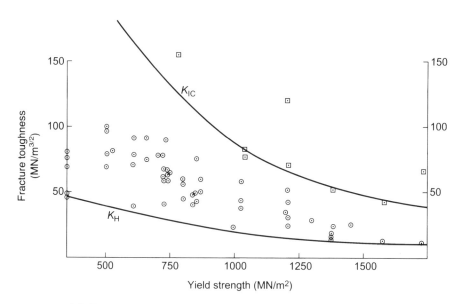

4.6 Fracture toughness of quenched and tempered steels. Data are from various sources.

growth is, initially at least, low, such that in welds, for example, it is easy to follow with the naked eye.

Hydrogen cracking associated with welding has initiated a number of catastrophic failures. The disbonding that led to the *Alexander L Kielland* disaster was almost certainly the result of hydrogen-induced cracking, as will be seen in the next section. One of the three instances of catastrophes initiated by a brittle fracture and discussed below was probably the result of hydrogen cracking in a weld. Hydrogen cracking was directly responsible for the explosive disruption of two ammonia converters during service. Details of these two failures have never been published, however.

Lamellar tearing

A macrosection of a weld below which lamellar tearing has occurred is shown in Fig. 4.7. The contraction, caused by welding, has opened up laminations in the steel in a region close to the fusion boundary. These laminations run parallel to the plate surface and are joined by a shear fracture which forms at right angles to the laminations.

The primary cause of this type of failure is the presence of laminar sulphide inclusions. When steel is cast, two main types of sulphide inclusions may form. The first, which appears during an early stage of solidification, is spherical and more or less retains its form when the billet is rolled into plate form. The second type precipitates as intergranular films during cooling. These intergranular films are malleable and roll out to a thin, plate-like form. They reduce the strength and ductility of the plate in a direction at right angles to the surface.

The formation of spherical sulphide inclusions is favoured by the presence of free oxygen, whilst the intergranular type is characteristic of aluminium-killed steel. The formation of non-laminar sulphide inclusions may be promoted in killed steel by the addition of calcium or rare earth metals. Alternatively, the sulphur content of steel may be reduced to low levels by calcium treatment of the iron upstream of the oxygen converter,

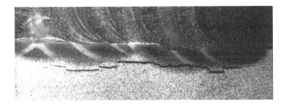

4.7 Lamellar tearing below a weld in carbon–manganese steel.

or by treatment of the liquid steel subsequently. By these various means it is possible to improve the through-thickness ductility of steel and thereby improve its resistance to lamellar tearing. Steel grades having a minimum level of through-thickness ductility are available and are used for critical parts of offshore structures.

It is known that the presence of hydrogen in weld metal, for example, because of the use of cellulose-coated electrodes, increases the risk of lamellar tearing. It may well play an essential role, since the fractures that join the laminations are brittle in character. Hydrogen cracks initiated at the tip of the lamination could well take this form.

There is another type of defect that is very similar in its general form and which is undoubtedly due to hydrogen. This failure mode first appeared in the Persian Gulf during the early 1970s and affected pipelines carrying moist hydrocarbon gas contaminated with hydrogen sulphide. Corrosion by hydrogen sulphide results in the release of atomic hydrogen, which supersaturates the metal with hydrogen. The hydrogen initially concentrates at the sulphide–metal interfaces and then precipitates, forming laminar cavities, which join up as in lamellar tearing and finally lead to complete rupture. Because the steel is supersaturated with hydrogen, the gas in these cavities may be at high pressure. As in lamellar tearing, cracks propagate at right angles to the laminations, joining those discontinuities stepwise. No catastrophes have ensued, but there was considerable disruption and cost when the problem first appeared.

Catastrophes resulting from the brittle failure of steel

The Liberty ships[7]

Two standard types of vessels were built from 1941 onwards in the Kaiser shipyards, the Liberty ships, which carried general cargo, and the T2 oil tankers. Both were fully welded, and for the time the speed of construction was remarkable; the first T2 tankers took on average 149 days to complete but by the tenth round of contracts, this time was down to 41 days. Large numbers were produced and they made a massive contribution to the war capability of Britain and later the Allies.

At the start there was virtually no experience of welded ships and there were some built-in stress concentrations, notably at square hatch corners, the end of bilge keels and at cut-outs in the shear strakes. These discontinuities were the origin of most of the serious brittle fractures. The loss rate became serious in the winter and spring of 1942–43 and peaked during the same period of 1943–44. The US ship structures committee later analysed the records and classified the types of failure. Class 1 included those where there were one or more fractures that endangered the ship or resulted in its loss. For the original design, the rate of Class 1 casualties was 4.3 per 100 ship-years, as compared with losses from all causes of 1 per 100 ship-years immediately before the war.

After the severe winter of 1943–44 the design was improved by reducing the severity of notches and by introducing a minimum of four riveted seams running the length of the hull and intended as crack arresters. With the improved design details the Class 1 casualty rate fell to 0.5 per 100 ship-years. The riveted crack-arresters were less successful; without them T2 tankers had a Class 1 failure rate of 1.9 per 100 ship-years, but with the riveted seams that figure fell to 1.2.

The other factor that became evident in 1943 was that the casualty rate was worse at low temperatures and in rough seas. So from that time the Liberty ships were, wherever possible, routed through calmer and less icy waters.

The impact properties of plate from some of the casualties were measured. It was found that plates in which brittle failures originated had a 21 J transition temperature of 15–65 °C with a mean of 40 °C. Such steel would undoubtedly have been notch-brittle during winter and spring in the North Atlantic. Improved steel qualities were developed soon after the Second World War and the incidence of brittle fracture fell. Weld quality was likewise improved. Some of the early brittle fractures were initiated by weld defects and particularly by cracks. The improvement in steel quality continues: in 1991 Lloyd's Rules included provision for 16 grades of as-rolled or normalised and 18 grades of quenched and tempered steel. All are impact-tested except the A grade, which is a general-purpose mild steel for use in non-critical locations. The lowest impact-tested grade calls for a 27 J transition temperature of 0 °C, the highest for an impact strength of 41 J at −60 °C.[7]

The Sea Gem[8,9]

This ill-fated vessel started life in the army. It was built in 1953 as a jack-up section of an aerial tramway (cableway) for the US Transportation Corps and operated as such during 1955–56. It was then mothballed until 1962 when it was declared surplus to US Army requirements. After being purchased by the French contractor Hersent, the hull was modified and it was used as a flat-topped barge in the Persian Gulf, under the name *GEM 103*. GEM was the Compagnie Générale d'Equipements pour les Travaux Maritimes, a joint subsidiary of the De Long Corporation of New York and Hersent of Paris. In the spring of 1964 *GEM 103* was towed to Bordeaux and re-converted into a ten-leg jack-up platform, using De Long jacks (to be described later). For the rest of 1964 it was used as a civil engineering platform.

At this time British Petroleum was assembling material for use on the newly discovered North Sea field and it was decided that *GEM 103* would be suitable for North Sea drilling subject to certain modifications. So the rig was hired by the contractor Wimpey, who remained responsible for maintenance, and then re-hired by British Petroleum.

The original hull was 300 ft in length, 90 ft in beam and 13 ft deep. In order to provide a drilling slot, a length of 100 ft was cut off the stern and a newly fabricated section 47 ft long was added. A heavy duty crane and the drilling derrick were mounted on the deck, together with other necessary equipment such as accommodation, a radio room and a helideck. Two legs were mounted in the new section, making ten in all, as before. The legs, which were 5 ft 11 in in diameter were cut and a new central length of 128 ft inserted, making them 220 ft in length altogether. The new part was intended to be that normally engaged by the jacks. Figure 4.8 shows the rig, by that time named the *Sea Gem*.

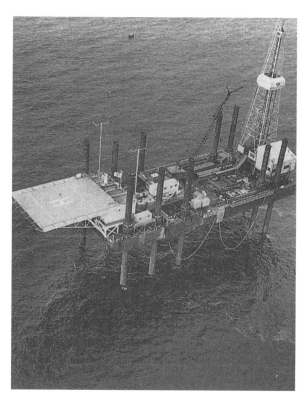

4.8 The *Sea Gem*.

During the construction period there was considerable discussion about the means of avoiding brittle fracture and in particular about the level of impact energy to be specified for the plate material. Eventually the figure of 25 ft-lb at 0 °C was established as the basic requirement; material not meeting this figure was to be normalised. Normalising consists of heating the steel to a temperature above the ferrite–austenite transition, say 950 °C, and cooling in air. This refines the grain and improves notch-ductility and impact strength. In fact, owing to an error in translating metric units to foot-pounds, the borderline level for normalising was 20 ft-lb at 0 °C.

It is not clear from the record whether any tests were carried out on the material of the original structure, which dated from 1952. Presumably not, because a failure would logically have required that the whole barge be rebuilt.

The De Long type D jacks (Fig. 4.9) consisted of a circular framework mounted on the deck which contained two sets of grippers. These were

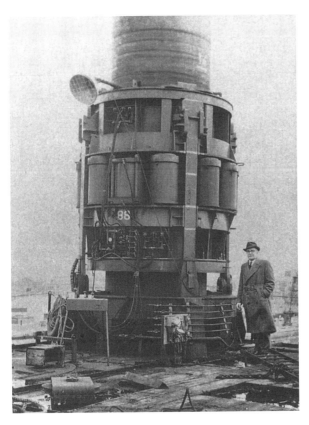

4.9 Type 'D' De Long air jack fitted on drill barge *Sea Gem*.

made of nylon-reinforced neoprene rubber and were forced against the leg by air pressure. The upper set of grippers was attached to the decks by four equally spaced tiebars. The lower grippers were connected to the upper set by 12 pneumatically operated cylinders (visible in the photograph) which were supplied with air at 350 psi by a set of four compressors. There were non-return valves that retained the pressure on the grippers in the event of a failure in the air supply.

To raise the platform the lower set of grippers remained fixed and the upper set was released. The cylinders were then pressurised, which raised the upper grippers and the platform by 13 in. The upper grippers were then applied and the lower ones released. Retracting the cylinders raised the lower grippers by 13 in so that the cycle could be repeated. To lower the platform the operation was reversed. Except when raising or lowering, both sets of grippers were applied. At all times the platform was suspended from the jacks by tiebars. The integrity of the structure relied, first, on the strength of the tiebars and, second, on the frictional force between the grippers and the legs. Operators were provided with carbon tetrachloride to clean off any grease and fine sand to improve the grip.[8]

The *Sea Gem* was towed out to the required position and on 3 June 1965 was successfully jacked up to the drilling position 50 ft above sea level. The sea bed was sand over boulder clay: the legs were designed to penetrate a few feet into the sand for better stability and this they appeared to do. Drilling operations proceeded without undue problems, the well head was secured on 18 December and preparations for moving the barge to a new location were put in hand. Such a move required at least 48 hours of favourable weather. Forecasts indicated that conditions could be right at the end of December and as a preliminary step the platform was lowered 12 ft. This was done by operating each jack individually. The lower gripper was released, the cylinders extended and the gripper applied again. When all jacks had functioned in this way, the barge was lowered one stroke by working all jacks together from the central control. The upper grippers were all released, the cylinders depressurised and the grippers applied again.

The accident

On 27 December the weather conditions were considered to be good enough to lower the platform a further 10 ft. The air temperature was about 3 °C and the water temperature about 6 °C with a force 5 wind and waves not higher than 10 ft. The jacks had proved to be in good order for lowering, but in view of the possible need to raise the platform if conditions deteriorated, the operator decided first of all to raise it by one stroke. This operation was conducted from the central control; the upper grippers were released and when the pressure at the cylinders had reached 300 psi, the forward end of the barge started to rise. At the full pressure, however, the aftermost jacks had not moved at all. The operator made a visual check, and then started to release pressure. At this point there was a loud bang and the platform lurched violently to port. This movement was suddenly arrested, probably because the port side legs jammed in their wells. The platform then righted itself and fell more or less horizontally into the sea. For the time being it floated, but the fall had caused a brittle crack to extend right across the bottom and water was pouring in. The wreckage remained afloat for 10–15 minutes, then capsized and sank.

During this time some of the crew showed commendable presence of mind and courage. Two liferafts were launched, both from the starboard side. Five men got into No 3 liferaft and 14 into No 1. The toolpusher, who is normally in charge of drilling operations and was the senior man on board, took command of No 1 raft. At the time there were ten men on the helideck or thereabouts. Mr Hewitt, the toolpusher, called on these men to come down and board one of the liferafts, but they stayed where they were. When the situation became too dangerous Mr Hewitt cast off. Even then he manœuvred the raft as close to the helideck as possible in an attempt to rescue these men, but was not successful. The liferafts were then paddled or drifted over to the MV *Baltrover*, a ship on passage from Gdynia to Hull, which had passed within sight of the rig when it collapsed. With some difficulty all those on the liferafts were taken on board this ship. All those who remained on the wreck died, including two who were rescued from the sea by helicopter but died later. During the initial phase of the collapse both the radio room and the *Sea Gem*'s one lifeboat had been pitched into the sea. The radio operator swam over to the lifeboat and got aboard, but died of cold.

The cause of the accident

The inquiry tribunal[9] had few doubts about this question: the most probable cause of the collapse was the brittle failure of tiebars on the port side of the rig. Moreover, most of the fractures of legs and other parts of the structure that occurred as a result of this initial failure were brittle fractures. Figure 4.10 shows the remains of one broken leg. The fracture is completely brittle.

The tiebars or suspension links, however, were the real problem. The form and dimensions of these members are shown in Fig. 4.11. They were flame cut from $2\frac{1}{2}$-in thick plate, nominally to ASTM A36 but possibly to

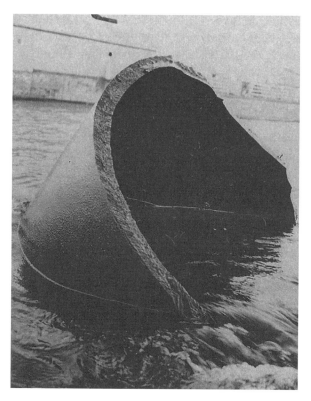

4.10 Fractured caisson of *Sea Gem*, 31 January 1966.

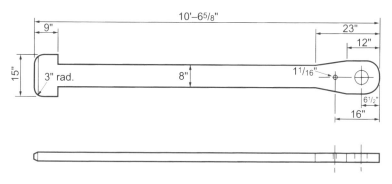

4.11 Dimensions of tiebars of De Long air jacks on *Sea Gem*.

an equivalent French standard. A36 is a structural grade of carbon steel with no special requirements for notch-ductility, the only concern of the designers being with its tensile strength. The jacks, including tiebars, were fabricated by the firm of Lecq of Douai, France in early 1964 when *GEM 103* was made. The material was not subject to impact testing or normalising.

There were a number of reasons why the Tribunal considered that fracture of the tiebar was the initial cause of the disaster. These were:

1 The divers' survey of the wreckage showed that tiebars on the port side were either missing or fractured.
2 One complete and six fractured bars were recovered, and all the fractures were brittle in character.
3 The temperature at the time of the accident was 3 °C, low enough for the steel to be in a notch-brittle condition.

In addition, survivors recalled that immediately after the platform fell, two or possibly three jacks were left attached to the legs.

There had also been a previous failure. On the night of 23/24 November a loud bang was heard and investigation showed that two tiebars on the No 12 leg had broken. These were replaced with spares within a few hours and there was no concern about the incident among those on board. After the loss of the *Sea Gem* the two links were examined by the UK Safety in Mines Research Establishment who found that the failures were indeed brittle and had initiated at a sharp corner radius at the spade end of the member (later measurements showed this radius to be 0.08 in). In addition, there were gouge marks in the flame cut edges and several weld runs where an attempt had been made to repair such gouges. The hardness of the heat-affected zone of these weld runs was excessively high compared with that of the original plate. The welds contained porosity and slag inclusions (Fig. 4.12) and cracks were found near the fusion boundary. One of the brittle failures was identified as having initiated at a weld.

It was also found that the pin holes were slightly elongated, indicating that at some stage the links had been stressed beyond the yield strength. The tiebars recovered from the wreck were examined in the laboratory of Lloyd's Register of Shipping and these all showed a similar feature. The reason for this apparent overloading has not been explained.[10]

Lloyd's[11] carried out impact tests on samples from the seven pieces of bar; the results have been averaged and are plotted as a transition curve in Fig. 4.13. The transition curve for steel from the *Alexander L Kielland* wreck is plotted on the same diagram to show how the notch-ductility of structural steel had improved in the 15 years between the two catastrophes. The mean impact strength of the tiebar material at 0 °C was 17.5 J, about 13 ft-lb.

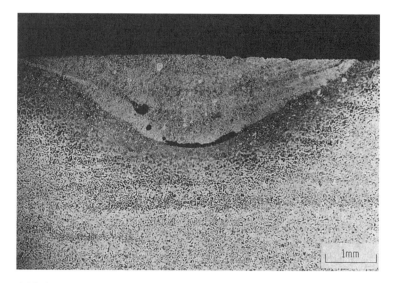

4.12 Section of a typical weld run on one of the *Sea Gem* tiebars.

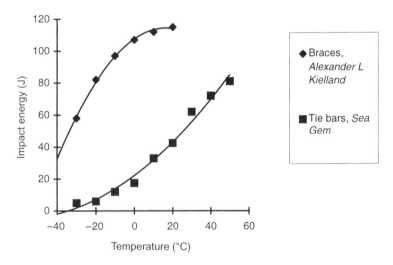

4.13 Charpy V energy transition curves: tiebars from *Sea Gem* compared with samples from braces of the *Alexander L Kielland* wreck.

These items therefore combined low notch-ductility with the presence of serious defects caused by surface weld runs which had not been heat treated. At the time of the accident, conditions for initiation and propagation of brittle cracks in the tiebars were present in full measure.

Ammonia tank failure[12]

Liquid anhydrous ammonia is used as a fertiliser. It is stored either at room temperature under pressure or at atmospheric pressure and maintained at subzero temperature. At a fertiliser plant in Potchefstroom, South Africa, the ammonia was stored under pressure in four 50-ton horizontal cylinders of the type known as bullets. On 13 July 1973 one of these bullets exploded whilst being filled from a rail car. An estimated 30 tons of liquid ammonia escaped from the vessel and a further 8 tons was lost from the rail car before the feed pump could be shut down. The air was still at the time of the spill and a large gas cloud formed, but within a few minutes a slight breeze arose, driving the gas over the perimeter fence and into a neighbouring township.

One man was killed instantly by the explosion. Others who were close to and in the direct line of the blast tried to escape but were overcome; two men managed to climb out of a storage tank and ran 25 yards before collapsing. The occupants of a control room about 80 yards from the explosion survived, including one man who was pulled inside with his clothes soaked in ammonia and covered with ice (ammonia chills sharply as it expands). They put wet cloths over their faces and after about half an hour were led to safety. Outside the factory, in the township, four people were killed immediately and two others died later. There were 18 deaths altogether, 65 people were treated in hospital and an unknown number by doctors outside the hospital.

At the time of the accident the tank car was filling No 3 and 4 tanks simultaneously. It was No 3 tank that failed and fortunately an emergency valve in the line connecting the two tanks shut and held back the contents of No 4 tank. The temperature of the liquid ammonia was 15 °C and the pressure 90 psi. The vessels were designed to British Standard 1515 for an operating pressure of 250 psi. There was therefore no question of the vessels being subject to an overpressure.

The failure occurred when a disc-shaped piece of metal blew out of one of the heads. Figure 4.14 is an end-on sketch of the failed head showing the outline of the disc. The points marked A and B are, respectively, the sites of major and minor repair welds, whilst C was the origin of the brittle fracture. There was no obvious cause of fracture initiation. The day was sunny, the temperature was 19 °C and there would have been a modest thermal stress due to the ingress of relatively cold liquid. The fracture itself was undoubtedly brittle; there was no measurable thinning of the plate and the fracture surfaces showed the typical chevron marks. The blank for the head had been made up by welding together two carbon steel plates 23 mm thick, one large and one small. Subsequent tests showed that the large plate had an impact transition temperature of 115 °C, and the small plate had

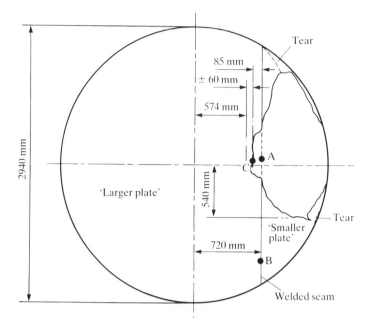

4.14 Brittle failure of the dished end of an ammonia storage tank.

one 20 °C longitudinal and 35 °C transverse. The large plate had a hardness of about 200 Vickers and a small or zero elongation in the tensile test. Clearly this plate (which is the one in which the fracture initiated) was very brittle indeed.

The cause of this extreme brittleness is not at all clear. The head had been made by cold forming the major radius and hot forming the knuckle at about 800 °C. It had not been heat treated subsequently and the vessel itself was not given a post-welding heat treatment because this was not required by the code. The steel had been ordered to a British Standard and the chemical composition conformed to requirements and did not show any peculiarities. Metallurgists investigating the problem suggested that the embrittlement could have been due to strain ageing following the cold-forming operation. However, many pressure vessel heads are made from similar steels in this way without disastrous consequences. Temper brittleness would appear to be a more likely cause of the problem. The impurities that promote this type of hardening are arsenic, antimony and tin, and such elements are not normally the subject of analytical tests. Thus a piece of susceptible material could escape detection and suffer embrittlement on cooling from the hot-forming operation.

The reason for the repair welding is interesting. The bullet was subject to a mandatory periodic inspection. The previous one had been carried out in late 1971. Normally a hydrostatic test was required, but the company obtained an exemption subject to an ultrasonic scan of the plate. The ultrasonic scan showed lamination in the larger plate of the dished head. Two areas of weld were scheduled for repair, either because of weld defects or because there were laminations close to the weld boundary. One repair (the one marked B in Fig. 4.14) was made satisfactorily, but the other (A) gave trouble and eventually there was a substantial repair area 8 in long. Finally, a hydrostatic test was carried out, but the head was not subjected to a stress-relieving heat treatment.

The residual stress field associated with the large repair weld was undoubtedly a major contributor to the disaster. The point of initiation was close to the repair and the brittle fracture formed a closed loop, which is a rare feature and suggests that residual stress was the main driving force for the crack. Internal pressure then projected the broken-out piece for a distance of forty yards: it finally collided with and ruptured an acid tank.

The owners of the plant (AE and CI; in earlier times, African Explosives and Chemical Industry) resolved that in future formed heads, completed pressure vessels and repair welds should all be given a stress-relieving heat treatment. They also decided to provide gas-proof rooms in hazardous areas.

This experience teaches yet another lesson: namely, that it is unwise to apply a test more severe than that originally specified for the equipment in question. Ultrasonic examination, in particular, is likely to expose defects which were not observable by visual or radiographic methods. Thus, a programme of unnecessary and undesirable repair work may be set in train. In the present instance the lamination, although undesirable, did not present a threat to the integrity of the vessel. The repair weld, by contrast, was a major contributory cause of the accident.

Generalities: catastrophes due to brittle failure

The two cases of catastrophic brittle failure described share two common features with the Liberty ships: the steel had a low notch-ductility at the operating temperature and serious defects were present which predisposed structural failure. In the case of the Liberty ships there were stress concentrations at the hatch corners, weld defects and fatigue cracks. The tiebars on the jacks of the *Sea Gem* had a sharp radius at the spade end together with surface weld runs that contained defects, combined with cracks and a hard heat-affected zone. The ammonia tank failure resulted from a combination of very brittle steel and a repair weld, giving a high residual stress field. In other words, the steel had been grossly misused in one way or another. Cases of pressure vessels that suffered brittle failure under hydrotest fall into a similar category: in almost all cases there was a combination of cracking with some degree of embrittlement.

There is an obverse side to this particular coin. The possibility of embrittlement caused by post-weld heat treatment in a furnace has been mentioned earlier. During the investigation that followed a vapour cloud explosion at an ethylene plant, samples were taken from two of the distillation towers that operated at subzero temperature. These were made of either $3\frac{1}{2}\%$ or 5% nickel alloy steel and impact tests showed that their notch-ductility was very low indeed. The subsequent history of these vessels is not known, but they had operated perfectly satisfactorily up to the time of the explosion. The ammonia tank at Potchefstroom had operated for four years with a dished end containing steel that had a transition temperature of 115 °C and a further two years with a severe, unheat-treated repair weld in the same dished end. Such experiences suggest that some structures can be very tolerant of embrittlement. In pressure vessels and piping this may well be due in part to the conditioning that the material receives during the hydrostatic test. The overpressure puts areas of stress concentration into a state of compressive stress and this provides a guard against subsequent failure at the normal working pressure. Proof loading of machinery and other equipment performs the same function.

Problems arise when some unexpected mode of deterioration or failure occurs, like the lamellar tearing that led to the loss of the *Alexander L Kielland* platform. Experience brings such problems to light and makes possible specific provisions against them. At the same time, the general improvement in the cleanliness and notch-ductility of steel that has taken place during recent years means that the probability of catastrophic brittle fracture is progressively being reduced.

There is one other matter concerning maritime disasters that deserves comment. It will be recalled that after the *Sea Gem* fell into the water, a number of the crew went up to the helideck and refused to come down and board the liferafts, even though urged to do so. In other disasters men behaved in a similar way. On the *Alexander L Kielland* they congregated on the highest point of the wreck and would not board the lifeboats. Launching these lifeboats was indeed a hazardous operation, but the alternative was worse. In the case of the Piper Alpha, men gathered in the galley, again one of the highest points and stayed there until the accommodation block fell into the sea. Some passengers on the *Titanic* were reluctant to leave the apparent safety of their quarters. A sizeable proportion of deaths was due to such conduct. Thirteen men from the *Sea Gem* lost their lives and ten of these were those who stayed on board the wreck. Eighty bodies were recovered from the galley of the Piper Alpha after the tragedy.

This human trait needs to be borne in mind when seeking to minimise the loss of life caused by disasters at sea. It could be argued that the problem is not that of providing a temporary safe haven, which is a straightforward design job, but how to persuade all the crew, not just the bold ones, to face the hazards and discomforts of the open sea.

Fatigue cracking

As well as being responsible for some major catastrophes – the Comet aircraft for example – fatigue failures cause a host of lesser breakdowns of plant and equipment and are responsible for a high proportion of service failures. It is, therefore, worth looking at the phenomenon in more detail.

Fatigue failure is an old enemy. It has been with us since the early days of the industrial revolution, when rotating machinery was first used on a large scale. A shaft carrying an overhung pulley could suffer many millions of stress reversals during its life and the earlier type of fatigue test, the Wohler test, employed a loaded rotating cylindrical specimen. From such tests it was determined that in the case of steel there was a fatigue limit, that is to say, a stress below which no fatigue cracking would occur, and that this limit was in the region of one half the ultimate tensile strength of the steel. Pulleys, gears and the like were (and usually still are) attached to shafts using drilled holes or keyways. Such discontinuities were found to reduce the fatigue strength. From the amount by which the fatigue limit was reduced, the stress concentration factor associated with the discontinuity could be calculated. Thus, in earlier times, it was possible to design machinery and equipment with some confidence by taking stress concentration into account and providing a safety factor on the ultimate strength. The advent of fusion-welded structures has radically changed this situation by introducing new uncertainties about fatigue behaviour. To explain how this came about it is necessary to consider the mechanics of fatigue failure.

A notable feature of fatigue cracks is that they occur at a stress below the yield strength and show no evidence of plastic deformation. The cracks propagate along relatively straight lines at right angles to the direction of the principal tensile alternating stress. On a macro scale the fracture surfaces show coarse striations, but when examined at high magnification it is often possible to find fine regular parallel ridges which are taken to represent the extension of the crack during the individual stress cycle (Fig. 4.15).

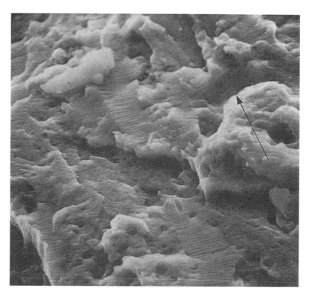

4.15 Striations on the surface of a fatigue fracture. The arrow indicates the direction of propagation (×1350).

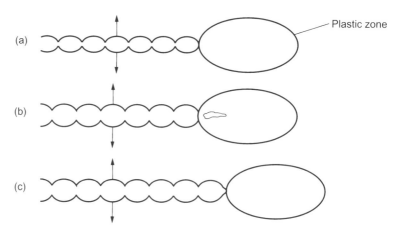

4.16 Fatigue crack growth: (a) start of half cycle, (b) incipient failure, (c) end of half cycle.

There is no generally agreed model for the fatigue cracking process but the presence of microstriations does indicate that it must occur progressively by steps. Figure 4.16 indicates how this may happen. The stress cycle is assumed to be from zero to a maximum tensile value. As the stress approaches its peak, a cavity forms in that part of the plastic zone in which the hydrostatic tension is greatest, immediately ahead of the crack tip. At maximum load the ligament between the crack tip and the cavity fails, the crack advances by one striation and the plastic zone reforms one striation forward.

According to fracture mechanics theory, the size of the plastic zone should be proportional to the crack length, that is to say, proportional to the square of the stress intensity factor K. So the crack growth per stress cycle should also be proportional to K^2, provided that the size of the cavity formed ahead of the crack is in proportion to the plastic zone size. Suppose that this proposition is correct. Then the crack growth rate is

$$da/dN = c(\Delta K)^2 \tag{4.2}$$

where c is a constant and

$$K = k(\pi a)^{1/2} \Delta\sigma \tag{4.3}$$

$\Delta\sigma$ being the stress range and k being another constant. These equations may be integrated to give

$$\sigma_f^2 N_f = \text{const} \times \ln(a_f/a_0) \tag{4.4}$$

Here a_0 is the initial crack length and σ_f, N_f and a_f are the stresses, number of cycles and crack length at failure. For test specimens having a constant width and constant initial crack size, the right-hand side of this equation is constant. A plot of log (failure stress) against log (cycles to failure) should give a straight line with a slope of $-\frac{1}{2}$.

Fatigue curves for three types of carbon steel specimen – plain, with a drilled hole and with a fillet-welded attachment – are plotted in Fig. 4.17. The log–log plot is indeed a straight line, but in no case is the slope of the curve equal to $-\frac{1}{2}$. In the case of samples with a fillet weld, there is likely to be a crack-line defect at the toe of the weld, as illustrated in Fig. 4.18. With such a configuration the fatigue life is occupied almost entirely by crack propagation, and the lower slope (about $-\frac{1}{3}$) simply reflects the over-simplified nature of the model proposed here.

In the other two cases it would have been necessary to develop an initial crack. When a metal is subject to alternating stress at levels below the yield stress, slip occurs across shear planes and after a large number of cycles this generates steps and eventually cracks at the surface. In such circumstances much of the fatigue life is spent in starting the crack. The lower the stress, the greater the number of cycles required to form a crack, so the fatigue life at low stress is increased to a greater degree. Hence the stress versus the cycles-to-failure line becomes less steep. Plots for welded joints other than transverse fillet welds lie between the two extremes and standard design stress figures are available based on the experimental data.

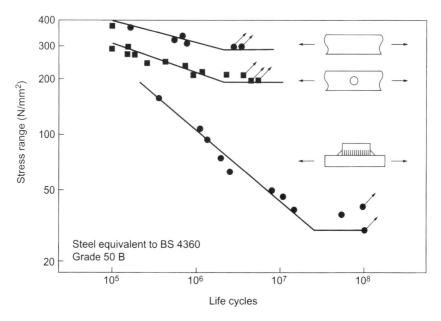

4.17 Stress range versus cycles to failure in a fatigue test for mild steel, plate with a drilled hole and plate with a transverse fillet weld.

Improving the fatigue resistance

One factor that affects the fatigue performance of welded joints is the presence of residual tensile stress. The effect of this locked-in stress is that when the member containing the joint is subject to an alternating stress that is partly compressive, the regions local to the weld suffer a completely tensile stress range, with a correspondingly greater risk of damage. As would be expected, stress relief is beneficial in those cases where 50% or more of the stress cycle is compressive. Design rules for structures (e.g. British Standard 5400) do not give any bonus for stress-relieving, but such heat treatment is used to some extent in vehicle construction.

A more general benefit is obtained by cold-working the surface around the toe of the weld in order to induce a localised compressive stress. Alternatively, the toe of the weld may be ground to reduce the stress concentration effect and to remove any crack-like defects. The effect of these two alternatives on the stress range versus cycles-to-failure curve is illustrated in Fig. 4.19. The ratio R indicated on the figure is that between the minimum and maximum stresses, and since tensile stresses are conventionally assigned a positive sign, this means that the stress range was entirely tensile.

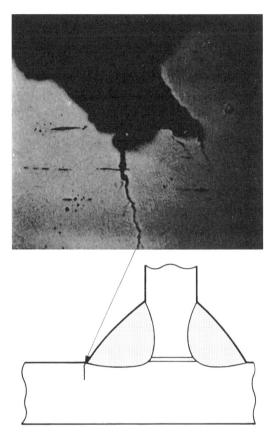

4.18 Fatigue cracking initiated at a slag-filled discontinuity at the toe of a fillet weld.

Cold-working for the test here recorded was carried out by hammer-peening, using a pneumatic tool. Taking the stress for failure at two million cycles as the measure of fatigue resistance, which is a commonly used criterion, peening more than doubles the permissible stress range. Although it is technically desirable, this technique has been little used in practice. One reason is the noise that it creates. In a typical case, the operator was (even with ear muffs) allowed to work for only 15 minutes in any one hour. The other matter for concern is the effect of cold-working on the notch-toughness of the steel. This is of little consequence for thin sections, but in the case of thick sections used for large structures, users have been reluctant to accept the risk. In fact, only a thin surface layer is affected and it is questionable whether there would be any real increase in the susceptibility to brittle fracture.

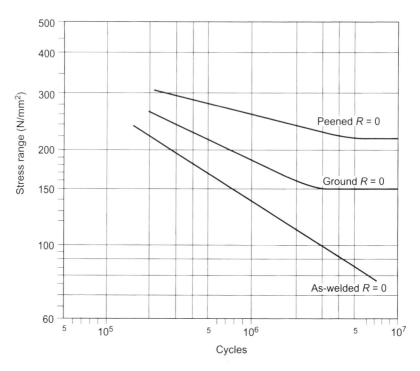

4.19 A comparison of the fatigue strength of fillet welds in the peened, ground and as-welded condition.

Recollections of the *Sea Gem* disaster still cast their shadows, however, and the more expensive and less effective technique of grinding has been specified for offshore rigs in critical areas such as the node connections. Grinding is done with a burr tool or a disc grinder – normally the disc grinder. Specifications typically require a groove of minimum depth 0.8 mm. Grinding has the advantage of being easier to apply and very much easier to inspect than peening. There are other methods of improving fatigue resistance, including remelting the toe area by means of a gas tungsten arc torch, but these have been little used in practice.

Service failures

Not all fatigue failures start at welds. A refinery manager well known for his dislike and distrust of contractors complained that his recently built hydrodesulphuriser was very noisy and at first this was thought to be a typical grouse. One day, however, an operator noticed a fine crack running around the inlet flange to the reactor. The unit was shut down and the flange removed; when examined it was found to be a millimetre or so from complete rupture. Further investigation showed that the refinery manager had in fact been right. The feed-effluent heat exchanger for the reactor had been so designed as to set up an organ-pipe or standing wave oscillation of fluid in the tubes. The resulting vibration had been transmitted down the transfer line to the flange, which failed at a sharp corner radius. Noise can indeed indicate an unsatisfactory state of affairs in process equipment.

Maddox[13,14] gives many case histories. Figure 4.20 shows two types of

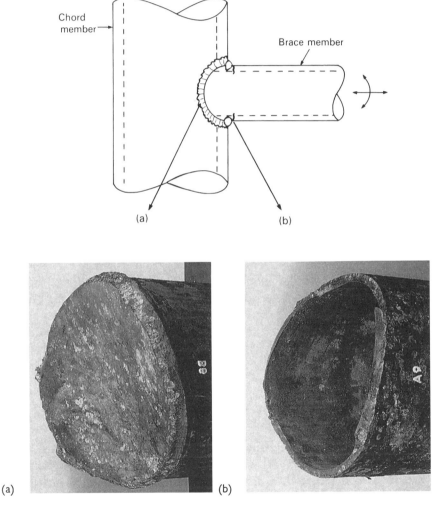

4.20 Fatigue failures of chord-to-brace welds in offshore structures: (a) from weld toe into chord, (b) from weld toe into brace.[13]

fatigue failure of a chord-to-brace joint in a fixed offshore structure. The brace in question was located near the surface and was therefore subject to substantial fluctuating loads due to wave motion. Horizontal movement of the chord gave rise to axial loads on the brace, as indicated in the sketch. This in turn initiated cracks starting from the toe of the weld on the chord side (photo (a)). Vertical movements on the other hand resulted in displacement of the brace and initiated a fracture through the brace (photo (b)). This problem was largely overcome by locating the braces at a lower level, but a few similar fatigue cracks have occurred in other areas, owing no doubt to the considerable height of waves in the North Sea.

Maddox also draws attention to the hazards caused by fabrication aids. One well-known example is the cleats that are welded to the outer skin of pressure vessels in order to align strakes or longitudinal welds. Most specifications require that such attachments be cut off, the surface ground smooth and tested for cracks, but whereas great care is taken in making procedure tests for the main seam welds, there is virtually no control over temporary attachment welds, which can provide equal and sometimes greater hazards.

Figure 4.21 illustrates two service failures that resulted from fabrication aids. The upper figure is a sketch of a section of a longitudinally welded tubular member which had been subject to alternating stress. The weld had been made on to a backing bar, whilst the backing bar itself was made up of short lengths of strip welded end-to-end, the pieces being joined by partial penetration welds. Fatigue cracks initiated at the unfused discontinuity in the backing bar and propagated through the pipe, as shown.

The other diagram shows a node area in an offshore structure. The braces are joined to the vertical member by butt welds and to make inspection of the root of these welds easier, a window was cut into each of the braces. Finally, the holes were repaired by welding in a closure piece. However, owing to the poor fit and an awkward welding position, the welds contained root defects. These propagated to the surface and although the cracks were found before any catastrophic failure occurred, repairs were difficult and costly.

Other types of fracture

Low-stress brittle fracture, which was a matter of such concern in the years following the Second World War, is no longer a large-scale problem. In recent years, however, there have been a few cases where steel structures have fractured, albeit under severe loading conditions, in an unexpected fashion. These are described below.

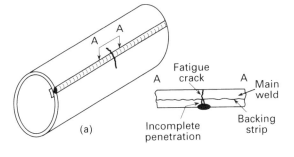

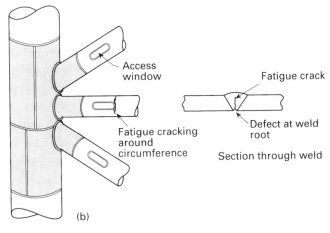

4.21 Fatigue cracking in service: (a) propagating from partial penetration weld in backing strip; (b) initiated by defect in root of single-side weld made to close up access windows in brace of offshore structures.[13]

The Alexander L Kielland *fractures*

Although the designers of this platform did not make any provision for the failure of any of its load-bearing members, there is no self-evident reason for its sudden collapse. Nor is there any obvious explanation for the manner in which the other braces fractured.

Figure 4.22 is a sketch of the members attached to column D of the rig, showing the location of the fractures. The numbers shown are those of samples that were taken for visual examination and measurement. In all cases the visual appearance was similar; the fracture surface was, apart from a few isolated areas, fibrous, and there was localised thinning which varied in amount from place to place around the circumference. The centre portion of brace D–E was recovered intact; examination of the ends showed that each had the same general appearance. Figure 4.23 shows the amount

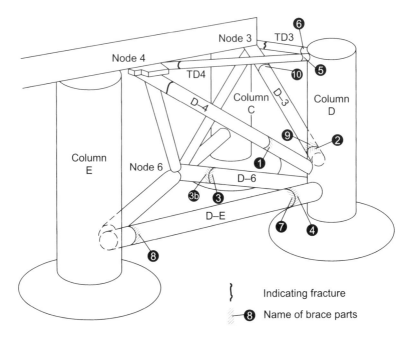

4.22 Fracture of braces around column D of the *Alexander L Kielland* accommodation platform.[15]

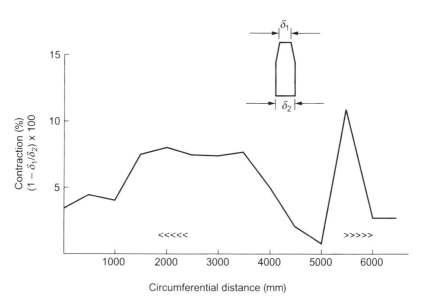

4.23 Contraction at fracture surface: sample 2 of brace D3.[15]

of contraction for sample 2 of brace D3, taken at one metre intervals. Also shown in this figure is the location of arrow or chevron marks, which occurred locally on most of the fracture surfaces.

From the description of these fractures, it is hard to evade the conclusion that they occurred as a result of axial tension and at a stress equal to the ultimate strength of the steel. There were two such fractures in each member, so it must also be concluded that they occurred simultaneously. The Norwegian investigators suggested that the second failure took place when the rig capsized and the projecting braces hit the sea bed. It is not easy to see, however, how a lateral blow could generate a fracture having the appearance described above.

Chevrons are characteristic of a running crack that has a curved front. They may be associated with slow (fatigue) cracking and also with fast brittle or ductile failure. It has been customary for those investigating brittle failures to use chevrons as an aid to finding the origin of the fracture and thereby to identifying the initiating fault. In the *Alexander L. Kielland* fractures only one such origin was found: this was a small area of cleavage fracture. There is no surprise here; these were ductile failures, which initiate normally in a cavity that has exactly the same type of surface appearance as the fracture in general.

When the brace D6 broke, there were two immediate consequences. First, the region of the column D around the connection relaxed. Second, there was a large release of energy following the relaxion of strain in the fractured brace. This would have been absorbed as vibration in the surrounding steelwork. Two such vibrations are probable. The first is an oscillation of the column, such that its cross-section became elliptical, with the long axis alternately in line with the failed brace and then at right angles to it. Consistent with this notion would be a compression wave in the adjacent braces. In such cases the motion would have been parallel to the long axis of the brace, giving alternate regions of tension and compression.

In order to generate the observed failures, three preconditions are required. First, there must be a stress distribution in the brace giving two peak tensile stresses at the points of failure. Second there must be some means whereby the end of the brace could be displaced by the distance required to effect the ductile fracture: a movement of several millimetres. Third, the energy released by the fracture of brace D6 must have been greater than that absorbed by the failures. Order-of-magnitude calculations suggest that these requirements could be met, but that the amount of strain energy released would only be sufficient to account for one pair of fractures. This would suggest a progressive collapse, the failure of one brace providing energy for the next fracture. Such a progressive series of brace failures is, indeed, generally thought to have occurred.

Whatever the merit of such speculations, it is clear that sudden, catastrophic collapse may result not only from brittle, but also from ductile failure. Ductile fractures were also found in steelwork affected by the Hinshin earthquake (see below) and these would, of necessity, have been fast fractures.

Earthquakes

Brittle fractures were found in welded structural steelwork after the earthquake at Northridge, California.[16] This earthquake occurred on 17 January 1994 in the Los Angeles area; it registered 6.8 on the Richter scale. The motion lasted 10–15 s, and the maximum ground accelerations were $12 \, m/s^2$ vertically and $18 \, m/s^2$, horizontally, which is very high for an earthquake. The air temperature at the time (4.31 am) was 40 °F, but much of the steelwork was enclosed so that its temperature could have been higher. There was much structural damage, particularly to concrete structures (Fig. 4.24). There were no deaths or injuries, however, and none of the structural steelwork collapsed. In more than 100 steel-framed buildings cracks were found at the joint between vertical and horizontal members. Figure 4.25 is a sketch of a typical failure. The crack originated at the root of the weld joining the lower flange of the horizontal girder to the vertical and propagated for a distance of about twice the weld thickness. In no case was either member severed.

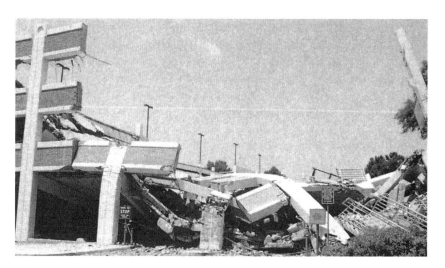

4.24 Damage to a concrete garage caused by the Northridge earthquake.

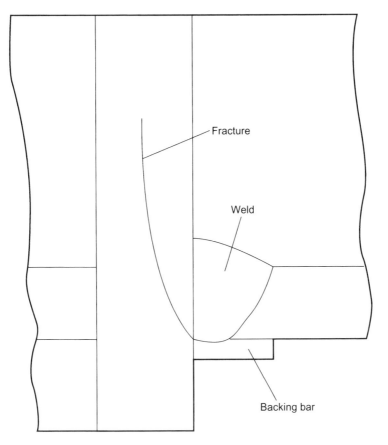

4.25 Typical brittle fracture in structural steelwork after the Northridge earthquake.[16]

As will be seen from the sketch, the welds from which the cracks originated were made onto a backing bar. Most welding engineers have a poor opinion of such joints, on the grounds that the backing bar may conceal and may even cause weld defects. Therefore, after the earthquake an improved joint was devised. The backing plate was eliminated, the root of the weld was removed and back-welded, and a fillet weld was made between the vertical and horizontal parts in order to reduce the degree of stress concentration. The improved joints were then tested and were found to be no better than the original type. So much for preconceived ideas about the demerits of backing bars.

The Hinshin Great Earthquake, which devastated the city of Kobe, Japan on 17 January 1995, shared some of the characteristics of the Northridge event. It measured 7.2 on the Richter scale, whilst the maximum ground speed was 1.04 m/s and the maximum displacement 270 mm. These are the highest figures recorded to date. About 5500 people were killed and 27 000 injured.

Most of the casualties resulted from the collapse of small wooden buildings. Only a small proportion of steel-framed buildings were severely damaged and a yet smaller proportion collapsed. Most of this damage was to buildings of two to five storeys. No steel-framed building higher than seven storeys collapsed. This record reflects, no doubt, the higher standards of design and construction required for multi-storey structures.

The pattern of damage generated by the Kobe earthquake was significantly different from that produced by other major seismic events. Its distinguishing characteristic was the large number of brittle cracks that appeared in the steelwork. These occurred at various locations: at beam-to-column joints, at splices in the columns, at the joint between column and baseplate and so on. Many were associated with welds, but some appeared at other points of stress concentration. Figure 4.26 illustrates one type of beam-to-column connection used in Japanese buildings. The column has a square box section, which is intersected by diaphragms at the joints. The flange of a short length of I-beam is butt welded to the diaphragms and the beam is bolted to the stub so formed. There are access holes (scallops) cut out of the web, as shown, and some fractures initiated at the corner of this cut-out.

The fractures fell into two categories; brittle cracks which occurred without any evidence of yielding (below-yield brittle fractures) and those where there was evidence of yielding or buckling in the vicinity of the crack. The former types were mainly associated with defective and partial penetration welds (these had been permissible under earlier building codes). In the case of butt welds, yielding before fracture was the norm. In a number of cases the cracks took a form similar to that observed after the

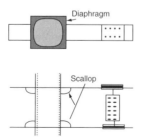

4.26 One type of beam-to-column joint used for the construction of steel-framed buildings in Japan.[17]

Northridge earthquake, as sketched in Fig. 4.25. They were short, the length presumably being determined by the duration of the seismic disturbance.

General comments

The three incidents described here show that under severe dynamic loading conditions (shock loading) fast unstable fractures may initiate and propagate in steel. Until the Northridge event, it had been generally assumed that in a severe earthquake any failure of steel frames would take the relatively benign form of bending or buckling. The appearance of brittle cracks is clearly a matter for concern. The circumstances giving rise to this phenomenon are clear enough, but a true understanding of the mechanics of such fractures is lacking. The possible role of elastic waves in fracture initiation was discussed in relation to the *Alexander L Kielland* fractures. Elastic waves are an essential feature of earthquakes and they could have a similar effect if the seismic disturbance is severe enough. Many questions remain unanswered.

Theoretical aspects of explosions

The catastrophe of war is fuelled by explosions, but in this chapter we are concerned only with those that occur in civil life. It is obviously desirable to know something about these phenomena, even though this will not necessarily point to any means of preventing them.

The behaviour of hydrocarbon–air mixtures

A high proportion of the domestic comforts of contemporary civilisation depend directly or indirectly on the controlled combustion of hydrocarbons. In the majority of countries (France is exceptional in this respect) most electricity is generated in power stations that are fired by coal, heavy oil or natural gas. Central heating boilers usually employ oil or gas as an energy source. The family motor car depends on controlled explosions of hydrocarbon–air mixtures for motive power. And for the present, at least, the rate of discovery of crude oil keeps pace with rising demand, whilst the known reserves of natural gas increase in quantity more rapidly than does consumption. It is in the refining of these essential sources of heat and power, and in transporting them from place to place, that the problems arise.

The Bunsen burner (Fig. 4.27) provides a good example of steady controlled combustion. A jet of methane gas comes out of a small hole

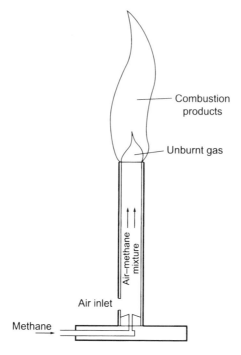

Combustion products

Unburnt gas

Air–methane mixture

Air inlet

Methane

4.27 Bunsen burner.

opposite the air inlet and the two gases mix. The mixture then passes up the vertical tube, where any turbulence is smoothed out. At the outlet of the tube the gas mixture burns radially inwards and, combined with the upward flow, this results in a conical flame front, inside which is the familiar blue cone of unburnt gas and outside is the feathery plume of hot burnt gas. All is in balance; the rate of advance of the flame front equals the rate of upward flow. However, if this upward flow rate is reduced too much, an instability may arise and the flame burns back down the tube and ignites the methane gas as it comes out of the small orifice. Any further burn-back is unlikely, however, because the flame would be quenched by the cylindrical wall of the orifice.

To ignite a hydrocarbon–air mixture two preconditions must be met. First, the mixture must be raised to its auto-ignition temperature. This is the temperature at which the combustion reaction is self-sustaining. Second, the heated volume must be large enough for the rate of heat generated by combustion to be greater than the rate of heat loss to the surroundings. In the case of volatile or gaseous hydrocarbons these conditions are easily met and a match or small electric spark is sufficient.

Deflagration and detonation

The conditions described above represent the steady combustion of a laminar gas flow. To achieve this condition it is necessary to provide a controlled rate of flow of the mixture. When a cloud of gas mixture is ignited there is no such control and the flame front advances in a disorganised manner. Two extreme conditions may be conceived. The first, which may occur for a short period after ignition, is a steady, relatively slow advance of the flame front. In the second extreme, the rate has become supersonic. The first condition is known as deflagration and the second detonation.

Detonation

This type of explosion occurs when a shock wave travels through a suitable material. A shock wave is a pressure wave travelling at a speed greater than that of sound. The material ahead of the wave is substantially undisturbed, and at the wavefront itself there is an abrupt rise of pressure. This pressure rise heats the material to its auto-ignition temperature or beyond, making the condition self-sustaining.

High explosives such as trinitrotoluene (TNT) behave in this way. A high explosive bomb consists of the main charge enclosed in a steel case, usually cylindrical. A tube or pocket running through the TNT (or other high explosive) contains a less stable chemical compound, the gain, and embedded in the gain is a substance that will detonate when struck or suddenly heated. The detonator creates an initial shock wave that is amplified by the gain sufficiently to detonate the main charge. At the end of this process the solid explosive has been converted into a mixture of gases at exceedingly high pressure and temperature. A gaseous mixture of hydrocarbon and air may be detonated in the same manner. Calculated initial temperatures and pressures resulting from such an explosion are about 3000 °C and 18 atm. Expansion of this hot compressed gas mixture takes place with high velocity and is preceded by a shock wave. Eventually the pressure behind the shock wave decays to atmospheric pressure and the shock wave becomes a sound wave. In the meantime, obstacles in front of the shock or blast wave will have been destroyed or damaged.

Early in 1941 the possibility of developing an atom bomb was being discussed in Britain and the USA. One problem was that although such a bomb would generate a large amount of energy, it would not produce the gases which result from the explosion of, say, TNT. Accordingly, Sir Geoffrey Taylor, an expert in fluid dynamics, was asked what mechanical effects would be produced by a sudden release of energy. At the time, his response was a military secret, but in 1950 the paper was declassified and published in its original form.[18] The prediction was, of course, that the mechanical effect would be the same as that due to a chemical explosion: a volume of air would be heated to produce a very high temperature and pressure and expansion of this volume would be preceded by a shock wave. Radiation effects were not considered in this study.

Assuming that the energy of the explosion E was generated at a point, the gas cloud would expand in spherical form. In this case the maximum pressure p_m behind the shock wave was calculated to be

$$p_m = 0.155 \, E/R^3 \qquad [4.5]$$

where R is the distance from the source of the explosion. When the first atom bomb was exploded, it was found that this simple expression predicted the results remarkably well. Comparisons with measurements of blast pressures produced by chemical explosives showed that the assumption of a point source caused the theoretical pressures close to the explosion to be too high, while at large distances the predictions were too low. In the intermediate range the trend was similar but the pressures calculated for the nuclear explosion were about half the actual pressures generated by a chemical explosion of the same energy. This is consistent with the idea that the gas produced by chemical explosions makes a positive contribution to blast pressure.

Figure 4.28 shows such a comparison, but in this case the multiplying factor in the equation has been doubled to give

$$p_m = 0.3 \, E/R^3 \qquad [4.6]$$

The measured pressures were made for a mixture of explosives that gave an energy release of 5024 J/g. The charge weight was 206 kg, giving a value for E of 1.202×10^9 J. Expressing the pressure p_m in atmospheres (1.013×10^5 N/m^2) and radius R in metres, this leads to

$$p_m R^3 = 3607.3 \, J \qquad [4.7]$$

At distances between 3 and 8 m the agreement between Taylor's equation (multiplied by 2) and measured pressure is very good.

The quantity $(E/p_0)^{1/3}$, where p_0 is atmospheric pressure, is called the 'characteristic length' R_0 of the explosion. The 'characteristic time' of the explosion is R_0/C_0, where C_0 is the velocity of sound at room temperature and atmospheric pressure. The characteristic length is an approximate relative measure of the radius from the point of explosion within which damage would be expected. For example, in the case of the mixture of explosives referred to above

$$R_0 = \left(\frac{1.202 \times 10^9}{1.013 \times 10^5} \right)^{1/3} = 22.8 \, m \qquad [4.8]$$

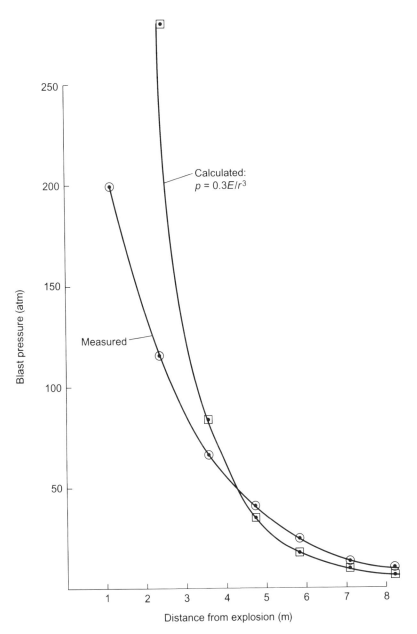

4.28 Blast pressure versus distance from explosive. One standard atmosphere is equal to 1.01325×10^5 N/m².

Extrapolation of a log–log plot of the measured values indicates that the blast pressure would fall to 1 atm at about 48 m distance. However, calculations of the extent of damage caused by explosions are notoriously unreliable and the best guide is obtained from empirical observations.

The detonation of hydrocarbon–air mixture[19,20]

One method of detonating gas–air mixtures is to enclose the gas in a plastic balloon and set it off with a charge of the explosive tetryl. Usually the volumetric ratio of hydrocarbon to air is such that enough air is present to oxidise the hydrocarbon completely; this is known as the stoichiometric ratio. The size of the charge required to cause detonation is a measure of the detonatability of the mixture. Much of the experimental work in this field has been devoted to methane–air mixtures, since methane is used and handled on a large scale. Figure 4.29 shows the results obtained by one set of investigators.[19] In this instance the figure for methane was obtained by diluting oxygen–methane mixtures with successively larger amounts of nitrogen and extrapolating the results to that corresponding to the composition of air. This gave an amount of 22 kg of tetryl. Others initiated detonations in stoichiometric air–methane mixtures with between 1 and 4 kg of high explosive. Even with these amounts methane is much the most

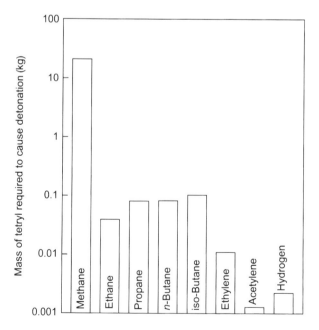

4.29 Detonatability of various hydrocarbon–air mixtures.[19]

stable of the hydrocarbon gases. This is in accordance with experience; there do not appear to have been any vapour cloud explosions caused by the release of methane. There have indeed been serious explosions at natural gas processing plants, but these could have been associated with the presence of propane. Confined explosions caused by methane leaks are, on the other hand, relatively common, and these will be mentioned later.

Relative detonatability is related to the chemical stability of the compound in question and this in turn is dependent on the ratio of the number of hydrogen atoms in the molecule to the number of carbon atoms. Carbon is quadrivalent, so that in methane, CH_4, all valence bonds are satisfied and the gas is relatively stable. At the other extreme, acetylene, C_2H_2, has a hydrogen : carbon ratio of 1 and is notoriously unstable. Ethylene, C_2H_4, is also easily detonated, and there have been serious vapour cloud explosions caused by ethylene emissions. Cyclohexane, which was responsible for the Flixborough explosion, has the formula C_6H_{12} and like ethylene, has a hydrogen : carbon ratio of 2.

Unconfined vapour cloud explosions[20]

Information on vapour cloud explosions is given by Baker and Tang[19] and in the Marsh and McClennan survey.[21] Other sources are listed in Baker and Tang's book on explosions. Accidents in which there was a large-scale release of gas were examined by Gugan,[20] for the period 1921–77. It was found that 60% had caused blast damage over a wide area, but it was considered that this damage was due to deflagration rather than detonation. In some cases the vapour cloud failed to ignite and in others the vapour burnt but did not have any blast effect.

It is not easy to account for the damage that does occur. In most cases the vapour cloud comes from the rupture of piping, less frequently from the explosion of a pressure vessel, and less frequently still because an operator left a valve open to atmosphere or made some similar error. Typically, the cloud spreads until it reaches a source of ignition, which may be an open flame or an electric spark. The steady burning velocity of a hydrocarbon–air mixture is about 0.5 m/s, whereas that of a detonation is calculated to be about 1800 m/s. There is no detonation source in a normal process plant, so how is it possible for the flame front to accelerate from 0.5 to 1800 m/s? At present there is no convincing answer to this question. The pressure build-up due to combustion does not in itself provide a mechanism; it is quite possible to envisage a pressure wave of constant height in company with a flame front of constant velocity. Turbulence of the flame front caused by solid boundaries has been proposed as a means of acceleration, but the vapour clouds with which we are primarily concerned often have no solid boundary. The type of damage produced by vapour cloud explosions is typical of that produced by a detonation blast wave. It must therefore be accepted that in some way, as yet to be adequately explained, ignition of hydrocarbon–air mixtures can result in an explosion.

Size may be a factor. It is perfectly safe to burn cordite in small quantities, but if a large amount is ignited it will explode. In gas–air mixtures, a finite time is required to develop the conditions for detonation and the larger the vapour cloud the more likely it is that these conditions will obtain.

One of the necessary preconditions for an explosion is that there must be reasonably good mixing of hydrocarbon and air. In most cases the escape is violent and the jet of fluid will be turbulent, such that the air will be entrained. In many cases there is then a significant period before the mixture ignites, sufficient for some diffusion to take place. It is very unlikely, however, that a stoichiometric mixture will be achieved and there is likely to be an excess of hydrocarbon. Consequently, the explosion energy is substantially less than that of the mass of hydrocarbon released. For actual vapour cloud explosions the proportion of material contributing to the explosion has been estimated to be between 1 and 10% of the total. At Flixborough, it has been calculated that of the 30 tons of cyclohexane released, only 5% exploded. The unburnt hydrocarbon is dispersed, or in some cases is consumed in a slow burn.

Confined explosions

Here there is no difficulty in supplying a simple explanation of what happens. Owing to the ignition of a hydrocarbon–air mixture, or sudden evaporation of a liquid, or some other cause, there is a rapid rise of pressure inside the container. If vents are provided, the peak pressure will depend on the balance between internal volume increase and rate of loss of gas through the vents. For example, if there is a gas leak in a house, and if the gas–air mixture is ignited, the internal pressure can build up to 8 atmospheres, at which pressure the house will be demolished. Normally, however, windows will be blown out first and, by acting as a vent, this may protect the walls.

Vents in the form of rupture discs are often used to protect equipment from the effect of an internal overpressure or explosion. Rupture discs are small in diameter compared with the container and are made of relatively thin corrosion-resistant metal. If the internal pressure exceeds a specified limit, the rupture disc bursts rather than the vessel itself. These items do not always work as intended. The reactor used for producing batches of resin for industrial coatings in a Cincinnati works was fitted with such a disc. Operators were using solvent to clean the reactor before putting in a new charge. However, there was some residual heat in the vessel, solvent was vaporised and the pressure built up to a point where the disc burst, releasing a jet of vapour. Unfortunately the reactor was located in a building and the vapour cloud accumulated in the roof until it hit an ignition source. The explosion wrecked the reactor building and damaged neighbouring buildings and stores at a cost of over US$23 million.

This particular episode was not unusual. The most common causes of internal explosion in process plant are excessive evaporation and processes that run out of control. For example, where a fluid catalytic cracker unit was being brought back on stream after a maintenance period, hot oil was introduced to a pressure vessel. However, the drain valve at the bottom of this vessel had not been properly closed and water had accumulated in it. When the hot oil hit the water there was an explosion and the vessel burst. The oil so released burst into flames and caused serious damage.

Internal explosions caused by uncontrolled chemical reactions take place from time to time, although they cannot be rated as common. One such occurred in a plant making a flame retardant material. This process unit, which was located in Charleston, South Carolina, was starting up after a maintenance period and operations had reached the second step of a batch process. However, raw material used at this stage was contaminated with water that had been used during maintenance. At the same time the water flow to the reflux cooler in the reactor had been reduced because of blockage. Consequently there was a build-up of temperature and rapid decomposition. The reactor burst, causing mechanical damage and spreading fire through the plant.

An internal explosion in a pipeline provided some useful lessons. This line was carrying fuel gas to an industrial area and it became necessary to increase the flow rate. Therefore the pressure in the line was increased, the planned level being within the capability of the pipe, but above the original hydrotest pressure. As the pressure was being raised, there was an explosion and a large fire, which fortunately did not cause any serious damage, nor were there any casualties. An electric resistance welded pipe from a reputable manufacturer had been used for this line and examination of the ruptured portion showed two significant features. First, the pipe had been dented at some stage, probably by a mechanical digger during the pipe-laying operation. Second, the initial failure had been a split along the centre of the weld and the adjacent length of pipe had split wide open, with 45% shear fractures. The most likely sequence of events was thought to be as follows:

1   The rise in pressure caused the dent in the pipe to pop out.
2   This event cracked the weld and gas started to escape, being ignited in the process.
3   Air was ingested into the pipe, causing an internal explosion.

Impact tests were carried out on the electric resistance weld, the V-groove being machined along the centre-line of the weld metal. The results were very low indeed and showed that the weld was almost completely brittle. There was no obvious reason why this should be so; the microstructure of samples taken from undamaged parts of the pipe showed no unusual features and were free of cracks and non-metallic inclusions. Samples of welds taken at random from electric resistance welded pipe of various sizes, however, also gave low values, not quite so low as the burst pipe but well below the normally accepted level. So the initial brittle fracture of the weld was not due to an extreme divergence from the norm, but rather to an unusual distortion resulting from the pressure rise acting on a damaged section of pipe.

Some ruptures are not followed by immediate ignition of the hydrocarbon. It is these that may cause vapour clouds to form and eventually explode. It is possible that ruptures associated with shock loading or (as in the case of the Piper Alpha accident) by impact will result in ignition, while other types of failure may not.

Underground explosions

Finally, it is only proper to make some reference, albeit briefly, to a problem that has caused many tragic accidents in times past and has claimed many lives; namely, explosions in underground workings, particularly coal mines.

The explosive in such cases is usually a mixture of hydrocarbon gases with air. The hydrocarbon is primarily methane and was known to older generations of miners as firedamp. It occurs in pockets whence it may diffuse into mine galleries and passages. At levels close to the earth's surface such a hydrocarbon gas may be produced by the decomposition of organic matter in ponds or marshy ground, where it is known as marsh gas or carburetted hydrogen. Methane-rich gas is also generated in refuse tips and on sewage farms.

Exceptionally, explosions may be due to a mixture of inflammable dust with air, but these accidents are more commonly associated with above-ground installations such as grain silos.

Methane–air explosions are of the deflagration type, but in the confines of an underground chamber are nevertheless devastating. The ignition source was, in times past, a candle or rushlight. The invention of the safety lamp by Sir Humphry Davy in 1815 was a major step towards improved safety in coal mines. Electric light is safer yet, but electricity may itself generate sparks and stringent measures are taken to minimise this hazard. Sparks may also be produced by steel implements, for example, if they strike rock, but this problem may be avoided by the use of non-sparking tools, usually made from copper-base alloys.

Many of the worst pit accidents (not all of which, of course, were due to explosions) occurred in deep mines. In spite of increased mechanisation, such mines have become less and less able to compete with oil and gas, on the one hand, and coal exported from more accessible seams in distant countries on the other. So the second half of the twentieth century has seen a sharp decline in the amount of deep-mined coal in industrialised countries. Although not very appealing to those immediately concerned, such developments have had an overall good effect on safety and conditions of work. This is one case where economic pressure combined with changes in technology (the evolution of the bulk carrier for example) have had a beneficial effect. This subject – the way in which technology affects safety – is discussed in Chapter 5.

References

1. Griffith, A.A. 'The propagation of rupture and flow in solids', *Phil. Trans. Roy. Soc.* series A, 1920a **221** 163–98.
2. Schardin, H. 'Velocity effects in fracture' in Averbach, B.L. *et al.* (eds), *Fractures*, Wiley, New York.
3. Robertson, T.S. 'Propagation of brittle fracture in steel', *J. Iron and Steel Inst.*, Dec. 1953 361–74.
4. Irvine, G.R. 'Analysis of stresses and strains near the end of a crack traversing a plate', *J. Appl. Mechanics*, 1957 **24** 361–4.
5. Boniszewski, T. *Self-shielded Arc Welding*, Abington Publishing, Cambridge, 1992.
6. Wessel, E.T. 'Linear elastic fracture mechanics for thick-walled pressure vessels' in Dobson, M.O. (ed), *Practical Fracture Mechanics for Structural Steels*, Chapman & Hall, London, 1969.
7. Smedley, G.P. 'The integrity of marine structures' in *Fitness for Purpose-validation of Welded Construction* (Paper 26), The Welding Institute, Cambridge, 1981.
8. Pratt, W., Lowson, M.H. and Rhodes, K.T.L. *Sea Gem Enquiry*, British Petroleum, London, 1966.
9. *Report of the Enquiry into the Cause of the Accident to the Drilling Rig Sea Gem*. Cmnd. 3409, Her Majesty's Stationery Office, London, 1967.
10. Lister, H.C. *The examination of some suspension links from the Sea Gem drilling platform*, SMRE Report Ref A608/543/01, 1966.
11. *Report on Tiebars T1 to T7*, Lloyd's Register of Shipping, R & TA No. 7984, 1966.

12. Lonsdale, H. 'Ammonia Tank Failure – South Africa', *Ammonia Plant Safety AIChE*, 1974 126–31.

13. Maddox, S.J. *Fatigue Strength of Welded Structures*, 2 ed. Abington Publishing, Cambridge, 1991.

14. Maddox, S.J. (ed) *Fatigue of Welded Construction*, The Welding Institute, Cambridge, 1988.

15. Anon *The Alexander Kielland Accident*, Norwegian Public Reports, Nov. 1981.

16. Skiles, J. and Campbell, H.H. 'Why structural steel fractured in the Northridge earthquake', *Weld. J.*, 1994 **73** (11) 66–71.

17. Toyoda, N. 'How steel structures fared in Japan's Great Earthquake', *Weld. J.*, 1995 **74** (12) 31–42.

18. Taylor, G. 'The formation of a blast wave by a very intense explosion', *Proc. Roy. Soc.*, 1950 **201A** 159–74.

19. Baker, W.E. and Tang, M.J. *Gas, Dust and Hybrid Explosions*, Elsevier, Amsterdam, 1991.

20. Gugan, K. *Vapour Cloud Explosions*, Institute of Chemical Engineers, Riley Park, UK, 1978.

21. Marsh & McLennan, *Large Property Losses in the Hydrocarbon Chemical Industries*, Chicago (published annually).

CHAPTER 5

How technological change affects safety

It has been demonstrated in Chapters 1 and 2 that accident rates, and the way in which they change with time, are determined by the relevant human population and are not affected by outside events other than major wars. Moreover it was shown that at any given time, the fatality rate due to road accidents varied very widely according to the productivity of the country concerned, in spite of the fact that the level of technological development of the motor vehicle is more or less the same worldwide. In other words, the loss and casualty rates are independent of the degree to which technology has advanced.

On the other hand, it would not be possible for those living in developed countries to perform their daily tasks if they were armed with only stone tools or, for that matter, bronze or cast iron tools. It has been proposed, therefore, that technical improvements should be regarded as an enabling factor, making possible improvements in productivity and, as a rule, in safety as well.

Matters are not, however, entirely straightforward. Suppose that when a new technology is introduced, the fatality rate falls exponentially from the start. However, at the same time the number of machines or vehicles increase. The combined effect is that the numbers of fatalities rises at first, reaches a peak, and then starts to decline. A simple mathematical expression that models this condition is presented in Appendix 1. The public is not in the least interested in the improved fatality rate; it knows only that increasing numbers of people are being killed. Such was the case in the early years of the twentieth century when increasing numbers of steam boilers were being installed in factories and laundries. The number of deaths caused by boiler explosions did indeed rise to a peak and then fall. The problem disappeared, of course, when electric motors, supplied by a central power station, became the prime movers in factories and elsewhere. The boiler explosions had one useful consequence, however, following a particularly unpleasant accident in New York. The American Society of Mechanical Engineers formed a committee to lay down rules for the safer construction of steam boilers. The work of this committee is of benefit to the engineering profession worldwide.

The development of the internal combustion engine has also produced a large crop of casualties and their incidence in developed countries, followed the same pattern as that due to boiler explosions. In Britain, annual deaths from motor vehicle accident rose from a very low number in 1900 to a peak of over 9000 in 1941, since when they declined to about 3000 at the end of the century. Although this is not very important in numerical terms, motor vehicles provide scope for the exercise of male bravado, as seen in the case of motorcyclists in Chapter 2.

On the whole, however, technical change is beneficial as far as safety is concerned, as will be evident from the historical details given below.

The role of the material

Steel

Developments in steelmaking

A number of the major catastrophes described in previous chapters were due almost entirely to the use of steel whose quality was inadequate for the job. Examples are the *Sea Gem*, the Liberty ships and the *Alexander L Kielland*. This is not to say that any of the designers concerned specified or used defective material knowingly; they were simply unaware of the potential problems at the time of the original construction. So it is of interest to see how far the intrinsic quality of metals, particularly steel, has improved and to consider how far this may affect safety.

During the twentieth century virtually all steel was produced by the indirect process; that is to say, iron ore is first reduced in the blast furnace to produce pig iron containing about 4% carbon, then the carbon content is reduced to less than 1% in a steel-making furnace or converter. The direct reduction of iron ore using hydrogen, for example, is technically possible and has been practised on a limited scale, but it requires a high purity ore, and is not generally feasible.

Before the Second World War a substantial proportion of the steel made in continental Europe was produced in basic Bessemer, or Thomas, converters (Fig. 5.1). This process was used primarily for iron that had been made from ores rich in phosphorus. The basic lining reacts with the phosphorus to produce a slag which can be used as an agricultural fertiliser. The converter was rotated so that its long axis was horizontal; liquid iron was poured in, it was then placed in a vertical position and at the same

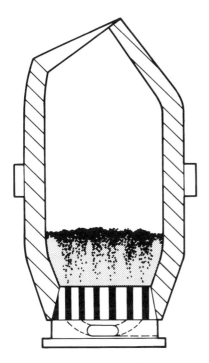

5.1 Bessemer converter. After the blow, the converter body is rotated through a little more than 90° to discharge the refined metal.

time air was blown through the nozzles or tuyères in the base. In this way the carbon could be reduced to the required level in about 15 minutes. The productivity of the Thomas process was high, but the high nitrogen content of the steel, picked up from the air injection, was undesirable and a number of modifications were introduced, such as blowing with a steam–oxygen mixture.

During the same period most British and US steel was made in open-hearth furnaces. These were large horizontal furnaces capable of handling 200–400 tons of iron. The bath was relatively shallow and heated by gas that flowed across the surface of the melt and then down into recuperators below. The carbon was oxidised by additions of iron ore, and in later years also by injecting oxygen through a long tubular lance. Productivity was lower than with the converter but it was possible to include scrap steel as part of the charge.

The third important steelmaking furnace at that time was the electric arc furnace. This was used primarily for remelting scrap.

Liquid metal from these furnaces was poured into ladles and thence into ingot moulds. Before pouring, a deoxidant could be added to the ladle. In continental Europe the steel was either fully killed or rimmed. In rimming steel, there was no added deoxidant and during cooling prior to solidification, carbon in the steel reacted with oxygen to produce an effervescence of carbon monoxide in the cooler parts near the mould surface. As a result the outer surface of the ingot was almost pure iron, but the interior was porous with impurities concentrated along the axis. Because of the porosity there was no shrinkage cavity at the top of the ingot.

In fully killed steel practice, aluminium was added in the ladle; this combined preferentially with the oxygen so there was no porosity and because of the contraction during solidification, a relatively large shrinkage cavity formed at the top. British and American steelworks favoured a semi-killed practice, where enough deoxidant (silicon and manganese) was added to prevent the rimming action, but allowed some porosity to form so as to minimise the amount of shrinkage. The economics of steelmaking were much affected by the amount of ingot that needed to be cut off to avoid defects in the rolled plate, and various other devices, such as heating or insulating the top of the mould, or pouring through a sprue into the bottom of the mould, were used to reduce waste.

After cropping the defective portion of the ingot, if any, it was reheated and rolled in a reversing mill. This consisted of a set of rolls with a roller-bed on either side. The slab was manipulated by pushers to and fro through the rolls until it had reached the required thickness. This operation was usually conducted in two stages. The ingot was reduced to a thick slab in the slabbing mill and then this slab was rolled down to plate thickness in a second mill. Alternatively, in the second stage the metal was processed continuously through a series of rollers (the continuous strip mill) and finally wound into a coil. It was expected that any pores or other discontinuities in the ingot would weld together during the rolling process but sometimes this did not happen and laminations in the finished plate were not uncommon. Typically, the steel so produced contained about 0.25% carbon, 0.04% sulphur and 0.04% phosphorus. It was tested for yield and ultimate tensile strength but only exceptionally for impact strength.

In 1948 the Austrian steel industry faced some special problems.[1] Iron made from locally available ore was not suitable for processing in basic Bessemer converters, so steel was made in open-hearth and electric furnaces. A substantial proportion of the output consisted of special high-quality steel that was exported and the supply of local scrap was small. There was a need to increase production and it was decided to develop a converter process using oxygen as the agent for removing carbon and other impurities.

Bessemer had patented the use of oxygen for bottom-blown, side-blown and top-blown converters in 1856, so the idea was not new. However, in the nineteenth century adequate supplies of oxygen were not available. Also, as it proved later, oxygen blowing results in high local temperatures, which destroyed the nozzles or tuyères. It was thought necessary to blow the gas through the liquid iron in order to get sufficient circulation. So it was decided to try top-blowing, bringing the tip of the nozzle either close to or just below the metal surface. Legend has it that during one of the test runs the lance broke well above the metal surface but the final result was not affected. So this arrangement became the norm.

The oxygen blow results in a violent bubbling action, which continues until the carbon content falls to about 0.05%. The liquid metal and slag undoubtedly circulate, but the cause of this circulation is unknown. Nonetheless, a new steelmaking process had been developed and by November 1952 the first unit was in operation. In Austria the process was called 'L–D', from the names of the towns, Linz and Donawitz, where the first tests were made. Elsewhere it is usually called the 'basic oxygen process'.

The metallurgical advantages were clear from the start. Impurities, particularly sulphur and phosphorus, were reduced to a low level without introducing nitrogen; indeed the nitrogen content of the original iron fell. Secondly, the operating time was short. Figure 5.2 shows refining curves for basic oxygen, basic Bessemer, acid Bessemer and open-hearth furnaces which illustrate this point.

The improvement in productivity was even more astonishing. By the early 1980s the vessel capacity had been increased to 400 tons, giving an output of 600 tons/hour, about 15 times that of a 400-ton open-hearth furnace. Naturally, the process was adopted worldwide and now most of the world's steel is made in basic oxygen converters.

One effect of the large potential output of the oxygen converter has been to make continuous casting a commercial possibility. Figure 5.3 shows the layout of a typical continuous casting machine. Liquid metal pours from a tundish into a water-cooled collar where a solidified skin is formed. The partially solidified strand then moves in an arc from a vertical to horizontal position, guided by rollers, and is eventually cut into slabs by flying shears. The advantages of such a method will be evident; the waste due to cropping ingots is eliminated and the slabbing mill is no longer required. There are also technical advantages. The steel is all aluminium-killed and there is no porosity and no shrinkage cavities. Therefore the risk of lamination is much reduced. Laminations in themselves have rarely caused any failures but, as seen in Chapter 4, the repair of discontinuities close to welds (which is required by some construction codes) can be hazardous.

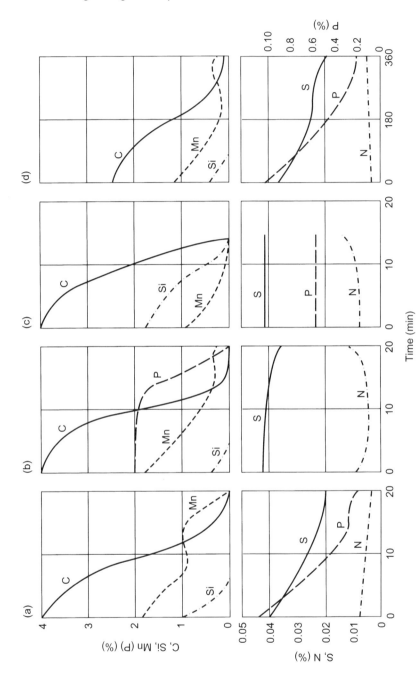

5.2 Refining curves for various steel-making processes: (a) basic oxygen; (b) basic Bessemer; (c) acid Bessemer; (d) open-hearth.

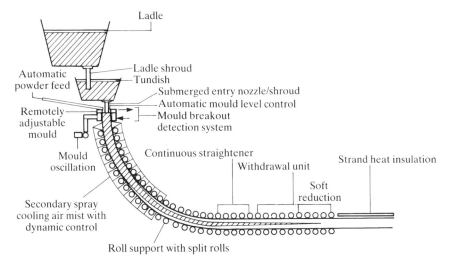

5.3 Continuous slab casting machine.

There have been other improvements affecting steel quality. In an integrated steelworks, iron from the blast furnace is conveyed to the converter in a torpedo car, which is an elongated ladle running on rails. Sulphur may be removed in the torpedo car (or in ladles) by treatment with magnesium, calcium or lime, whilst phosphorus can be removed using a basic oxidising slag. By such means it is possible to produce an iron with 4% carbon, 0.005% sulphur and 0.015% phosphorus. These values may be lowered still more by treatment after the oxygen converter. So it has become commercially possible to make a clean steel free from the laminar defects which reduce the through-thickness ductility of plates.

Finally, there have been advances in rolling mill practice. The objective of these developments has been to produce a steel that is fine grained in the as-rolled condition. Fine grain is normally associated with good notch-ductility and a low ductile–brittle transition temperature, combined with increased yield strength. In hot rolling, steel is subject to deformation at high temperature. By controlling this operation it is possible to arrive at the required mechanical properties.

The first steps in this direction were taken in some European mills in the late 1950s, where rolling was continued below the austenite–ferrite transition temperature. This did indeed have the effect of producing a fine grain, but it also developed a banded structure and elongated the sulphides, such that the material was subject to a laminar weakness. Subsequent developments have been directed towards controlling the operation at temperatures above the transition. The operation is known as 'thermomechanically controlled rolling' and it has many permutations and combinations. To take an example: when rolling is carried out at temperatures above 950 °C, the austenite grains are broken down by the mechanical treatment and subsequently new grains are formed and start to grow. By allowing the optimum time for recrystallisation after the final rolling pass in this temperature range, a suitably fine austenite grain size is obtained and eventually this structure transforms to give a fine ferrite grain size. In practice, rolling continues at temperatures below 950 °C and above the transition temperature to obtain further refinement. Figure 5.4 and Table 5.1 show some of the variations that have been used in the production of the Japanese steel HT50. This is a high-tensile steel (ultimate strength about $500\,N/mm^2$) used for welded constructions such as large storage spheres. The transition temperatures are very low indeed. HT50 is a special steel, but the technique is applicable also to lower-tensile grades.

It will be seen in Table 5.1 that small amounts of the elements niobium, titanium and vanadium have been added to some of the steels. These are known as microalloying additions and they act in various ways to refine grain and increase strength. Titanium, in combination with nitrogen, restricts the growth of austenite grains in the temperature range 1050–1100 °C. Niobium raises the recrystallisation temperature of austenite. Both these additions have the effect of reducing the grain size of the steel. Vanadium has only a modest grain-refining effect but increases the tensile properties by precipitation-hardening at temperatures below about 700 °C.

The overall result of such developments is that steelmakers can produce material of higher tensile strength and lower ductile–brittle transition temperatures at a relatively modest increase in cost. They have also resulted in an improvement in the quality of ordinary grades of carbon steel. Figure 4.13 shows a comparison between steel made in the 1960s with that made in the late 1970s. There is a reduction in the 27 J Charpy transition temperature of about 50 °C. Since that time quality has improved still further.

The effect of improved steel quality

It is unlikely that any of the catastrophic failures of steel structures described in Chapters 3 and 4 would have occurred had steel of 1990s quality been used, except perhaps for the case of the *Sea Gem*, where the damaging effect of surface weld runs on the tiebars could have been an overriding factor. This does not, of course, mean that the danger of such failures has been eliminated. Brittle fracture of steel having good notch-ductility is still possible under impact loading and where a fatigue crack

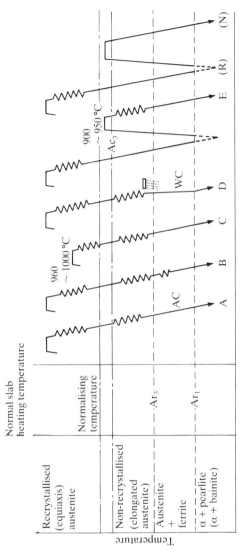

5.4 Controlled rolling of Japanese HT50 steel: thermal cycle. AC, air cooled; WC, water cooled; A, controlled rolling in γ region; B, controlled rolling also in γ and δ regions (separation); C, controlled rolling, low slab temperature and Ca–Ti; D, controlled rolling and water cooling; E, controlled rolling with reheating just over Ac₃; (R), as-rolled; (N), normalising.

Table 5.1 Controlled rolling of Japanese HT50 steel: mechanical properties

Rolling programme	Chemical composition (%)									CE (IIW)	YP (N/mm²)	UTS (N/mm²)	Elongation (%)	VE −40°C (J)	50% VTrs (°C)	Drop-weight (°C)	Grain size ASTM
	C	Si	Mn	P	S	Nb	V	Ti	Ni								
A	0.12	0.32	1.36	0.015	0.006	0.019	–	0.013	–	0.36	432	504	29	245	−91	−50	7–9
B	0.13	0.36	1.42	0.02	0.003	–	–	–	–	0.37	368	526	31	139	−92	−95	8–11
C	0.06	0.22	1.32	0.01	0.001	–	0.04	0.01	0.26	0.31	392	471	40	294	−125	−100	11–12
D	0.12	0.27	1.13	0.016	0.004	–	–	–	–	0.31	362	493	30	288	−71	−45	7–9
E	0.05	0.31	1.39	0.019	0.004	0.03	0.05	–	–	0.29	385	469	34	110	−97	−100	11–12
As-rolled	0.13	0.25	1.37	0.013	0.007		REM	0.035		0.36	420	530	22	200	−42	−10	4–6
Normalised											360	500	27	270	−80	−35	6–7

CE = carbon equivalent, YP = yield point, UTS = ultimate tensile strength, VE = impact energy, 50% VTrs = temperature for 50% fibrous fracture, REM = rare earth metals.

has been allowed to grow to an excessive length. Fatigue failure remains no more but no less a threat than in times past. It is not possible to produce a metal that will be immune to fatigue cracking. Avoiding such failures is not a materials problem, but rather a question of careful attention to detail at the design stage, combined with inspection during service. In this connection it is profitable to apply egalitarian principles. Designers are apt to designate particular areas in a structure – the nodes in the case of an offshore tubular construction, for example – as being 'critical'. Under fatigue loading conditions, however, all loaded joints, and particularly welded joints, must be given equal consideration.

It should be noted that good notch-ductility does not make a structure immune to sudden collapse. The *Alexander L Kielland* was made of good quality, notch-ductile steel. However, had this not been so, and had the steel been as brittle as that of the *Sea Gem*, it would have made little difference to the outcome. The important point is to use all means to avoid the type of failure that could give rise to such shock loads.

Aluminium

The problems that are so dominant in the use of steel, such as the embrittling effects of the common impurities, sulphur and phosphorus, and the transition to a brittle form at low temperature, do not exist in the case of aluminium. In order to extract aluminium, the oxide ore bauxite is dissolved in molten cryolite (sodium aluminium fluoride), and the solution is electrolysed. This process will only operate satisfactorily if the bauxite is of high purity. This means that the total impurity content should not exceed 0.5%, and the contaminants, mostly iron and silicon, do not have any embrittling effect. Thus there was not much to be done by way of improving the method of extraction. Most of the significant alloy development took place in the early days. The patents for the electrolytic extraction process were granted in 1886 and the age-hardening alloy Duralumin was invented by Alfred Wilm in 1909. Duralumin was a $3\frac{1}{2}$% copper $\frac{1}{2}$% magnesium alloy which, with minor additions, was used for constructing the Comet aircraft and is still in use today as alloy 2024. The fact that Comets suffered catastrophic brittle failures was not due to any deficiency of the material. As far as is known, there have been no subsequent failures of this type and the fracture toughness of aluminium alloys is not a matter for concern.

The introduction of the argon-shielded tungsten arc welding of aluminium just after the Second World War was a major advance. It is applicable to non-age-hardenable aluminum–magnesium alloys, which are employed on a large scale in the construction of ship superstructures and for offshore accommodation modules. It is applied on a more limited scale to medium-strength heat-treatable alloys of the aluminium–magnesium–silicon type. The high-strength precipitation-hardened alloys are generally regarded as unsuitable for fusion welding, in part owing to their susceptibility to liquation cracking. Friction stir welding (a solid phase process) is not subject to this defect and has been used in the fabrication of a small passenger jet aircraft, the *Eclipse*. In the prototype, which flew successfully in 2004, 60% of the joints were made by friction stir welding.

Air transport

The fact that so many aircraft accidents are ascribed to pilot error suggests that navigational aids and similar devices should be high on the list of air safety programmes. So this is an important subject and it will be covered separately in a later section. First, however, it is necessary to look at the development of aeroplanes in general.[2]

One of the pioneers of manned flight was Sir George Cayley. Cayley established the basic design and layout of an aircraft and the essential requirements for stability. In 1853 he built a glider and this made a brief but successful flight, piloted by his coachman. In Germany Otto Lilienthal designed and constructed numbers of gliders and made over 2000 flights before being killed in a crash in 1896. It was clear at that time, however, that no contemporary engine had the power-to-weight ratio which would make powered flight possible. The situation changed with the advent of the internal combustion engine. The Wright brothers made their first flight in December 1903 (Fig. 5.5). Their success was somewhat against the odds because the engine (which they made themselves) had a low power-to-weight ratio even for that time, and there was no tail or rudder.

There was more general interest in aeronautics in France than in America in those years and in January 1908 Henri Farman flew his own design of aircraft. In the summer of that year Wilbur Wright gave demonstrations in France of his pusher-type plane, creating great interest. Nearly all subsequent developments, however, followed Cayley's principles, using either tractor or pusher propellers. Blériot pioneered a tractor-type monoplane and in July 1909 flew it across that stretch of water known on one side as the English Channel and on the other as *la Manche*. This was a dramatic achievement and made Blériot one of the immortals of flying.

The same year saw the introduction of the French Gnome engine. This was a rotary machine; that is to say, the crankshaft was stationary and the air-cooled cylinders together with the propeller rotated around it. The Gnome was very successful and was used in many of the military aircraft produced during the First World War.

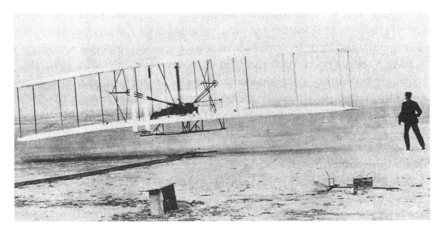

5.5 The Wright Flyer: first to achieve controlled powered flight on 17 December 1903.

The war provided a considerable impetus to aircraft construction. It has been estimated that in 1914 there were about 5000 aircraft worldwide, whilst in 1918 this number had risen to 200000. They were used for observation and as bombers, and light, fast fighter aircraft were produced to shoot down the bombers. The bombers were in many cases adapted for use as passenger planes after the war; indeed, custom-built civil aircraft did not appear until the 1920s and even then their design was greatly influenced by their military predecessors.

Before 1914, air travel was uncomfortable and unreliable. Only a few operators were brave enough to try to provide scheduled flights and these were usually for mail. There were aircraft, however, on the London–Paris route. The hazard for passengers was not so much that of being killed in a crash, but landing in a muddy field far from their destination.

After the war, aircraft, and particularly the engines, became much more reliable and regular passenger services became a practical possibility. In the summer of 1919 charter flights were operating between London and Paris and (in Germany) between Dessau and Weimar. Continental European airlines were subsidised by governments. This led eventually to the emergence of national airlines such as Lufthansa, Sabena, KLM and Air France. In Britain this was not the case at first, but in 1921 the operators refused to fly unless a subsidy was provided; this stance led to the formation of Imperial Airways in 1924. In the USA there was no such immediate post-1918 development; aircraft were used primarily for mail. The railroads offered a long-distance service which was safer, more comfortable, more reliable and cheaper than air travel, so initially there was not much incentive for airlines. However, in 1929 the Kelly Mail Act allowed the carriage of mail by private operators on scheduled services. Growth was then swift; by 1930 there were 40 small airlines carrying an annual total of 160 000 passengers. The big carriers such as American Airways, Pan American, Delta and TWA came into being during this period. Competition between airlines placed fresh demands on the aircraft manufacturers and helped to develop the design and construction of larger and safer airliners.

The pre-jet age

Early aircraft were made of wood, wire and fabric (Fig. 5.6). The flight surfaces were formed by stretching cloth over wood and wire frames and then doping the cloth. These covers did not constitute a major weakness as they did on airships, but occasionally they would disintegrate with disastrous consequences. Metal was, of course, more reliable, but although the first all-metal airplane, the Junkers F 13, was made in 1919, this type of construction did not become the norm until the late 1930s. Between these dates all sorts of materials were used. The original wood frame was in some cases replaced by high-tensile steel tubing such as AISI 4340, joined together by oxyacetylene or arc welding. Eventually the frame

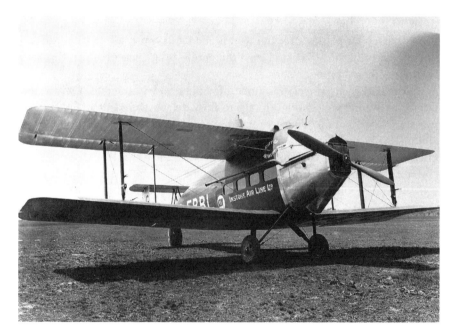

5.6 The Vickers Vulcan passenger aircraft. It cruised at 90 mph and had a range of 360 miles, carrying 8 passengers. The fuselage was made of plywood.

structure was replaced by a stressed skin with stiffeners, as in the case of the de Havilland Comet described in Chapter 3.

Biplanes predominated in the early days because for any given weight they are easier to design and build than are monoplanes. By the late 1930s, however, most civil aircraft were multi-engined, stressed skin all-metal monoplanes. This general type of design has predominated ever since. So far as material is concerned, an exception was the de Havilland DH 91, the fuselage of which was made of a plywood/balsa/plywood sandwich. The wartime 'Mosquito' night fighter was also made of wood, but these two are probably the last examples of non-metal aircraft.

The interwar years were the days of the flying boats. The advantages of these machines were that they required no landing strip or airport and they had a long range. Imperial Airways operated flying boats on its eastern routes and just prior to the Second World War started a transatlantic service, refuelling the seaplane in the air from a tanker aircraft. Dornier operated mail flights across the South Atlantic with Weil flying boats. The boats landed astern of a depot ship and were hoisted aboard and refuelled. Then they were launched by catapult over the bows to complete the last leg of the journey. Other flying boats operated in a more sedate manner and provided relatively luxurious conditions.

The Second World War had remarkably little effect on aircraft design; civilian craft were adapted for military use rather than the other way around. It did, however, accelerate the production of a viable gas turbine engine. The possibility of such a machine had been known since the early years of the century, but its realisation had to await the development of alloys (the nickel-base superalloys) capable of resisting the severe conditions to which the blades and disc were exposed. A Heinkel HE 178 aircraft powered by a gas turbine flew in August 1939. In Britain, Frank Whittle had run a prototype in 1937 and then, as war approached, received massive government backing. In fact, neither side made much use of gas turbine engines during the war and it was left to civil aircraft designers to employ them on a large scale.

In the late 1930s and in the early post-1945 period American producers dominated the field of long-distance aircraft. First was the Douglas DC3 (Fig. 5.7), which by 1939 was carrying 90% of airline passengers. The DC3 was a twin-engined all-metal monoplane which, in terms of numbers, was one of the most successful aircraft ever built. The later development, the DC4, had important innovations; the cabin was pressurised for high altitude flight and the wing structure incorporated multiple spars such that if a fatigue crack developed, enough load-bearing members would remain to prevent a catastrophic failure. The DC4 could carry 60 passengers, twice the capacity of the DC3.

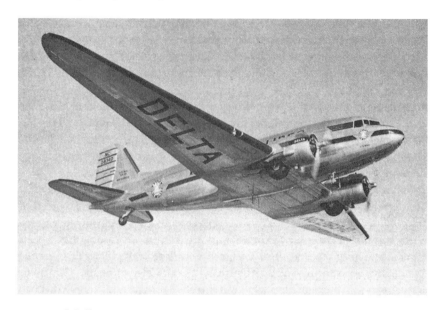

5.7 The Douglas DC3, one of the most successful aircraft ever built.

Thus, at the end of the war, there were a number of aircraft adaptable for civil use, including the DC4, the Lockheed Constellation and the Boeing Stratocruiser, which were designed for long-distance operations, flying at 200 mph or more, and high enough to be above the weather. Safety, reliability and comfort had been enormously improved in a remarkably short period.

Jet age

The jet age was inaugurated by the setting up of regular transatlantic services in the late 1950s with the Comet IV and Boeing 707. Both speed and range increased dramatically. The cruising speed of the Boeing 707 is about 600 mph, compared with 315 mph for the DC6. The Comet and the Boeing 707 had turbo-jet engines, in which thrust is obtained by ejecting gas from the rear of the engine. Numbers of aircraft in the early years of the jet age, however, used the gas turbine engine to rotate a propeller. This variant did not survive very long, however.

Comet IV and the original Boeing 707 were relatively small planes; the original Comet 1A carried 44 passengers. Boeing jets grew fairly rapidly; the 707-320C took 219 passengers. Then the 747, which came into operation in the early 1970s, could take nearly 500 passengers; the Lockheed Tristar took 400 and the European Airbus took 375. These large numbers made for uncomfortable journeys. The optimum was probably reached with the Vickers VC10, which had rear-mounted turbo-jet engines and flew quietly and smoothly with a complement of not more than 150 passengers.

Jet engines provide more than just increased speed and cruising height. Not only does greater power mean inherently greater safety in take-off, for example, but there are also other spin-offs. One of the most serious risks that aircraft face in cold weather is icing. Ice may build up on the leading edges of wings and tailplane, adding weight and making the plane difficult to control. Early de-icing devices included hollow rubber mouldings that were pulsated with compressed air in order to break off the ice, but these could be overwhelmed if conditions were really bad. Jet engines provided a virtually unlimited supply of hot air that could be fed to the leading edges so that the ice did not adhere.

Finally, there was the supersonic Concorde (Fig. 5.8), which first flew in 1969, had a cruising speed of 1354 mph and a passenger capacity of just over 100. The sonic boom was a severe disadvantage, such that the aircraft could only reach its full cruising speed over the sea or over uninhabited

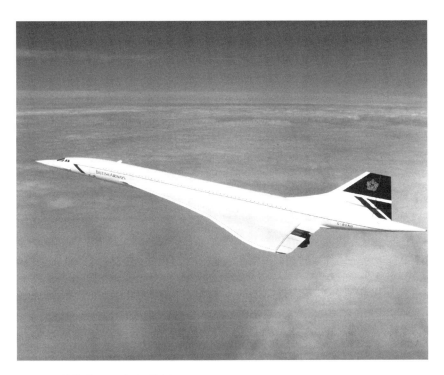

5.8 Concorde in flight.

country. Operating costs were high and although a more economic version is possible, it is doubtful whether this will be built, at least in the near future. Although this looks like a dead end, Concorde pioneered some sophisticated techniques, such as full electrical controls, which have had a positive influence on aircraft safety and it is one of the most beautiful aircraft ever designed.

Throughout this history of rapid development and change, the materials of construction have, on the whole, altered very little. The first all-metal aeroplane was made in 1919 using Duralumin and most aircraft flying today are built of the same or similar age-hardening aluminium alloys. A recent advance has been the introduction of aluminium–lithium alloys, which are lighter. Some supersonic military aircraft have a titanium skin, but this metal is still too costly for civil planes. Carbon fibre-reinforced plastic has found a limited use, for example, for the rudders of the Airbus 300 and 600, and glass-reinforced plastic may be employed for lightly stressed parts. Large changes in materials and basic format are unlikely in the near future. More development is possible in electronic control, as discussed below.

Control systems

These systems fall into one of several categories. The first comprises the means by which cockpit controls activate the moving parts such as ailerons and rudder. Second, there are automatic pilots. Then there are instrument landing techniques: aids to landing in bad weather. Air traffic control is a fourth area and finally there are systems that inspect for, and report, faults in other systems – very much a product of the electronic age. The techniques that fall into such categories are all intended to improve safety.

Autopilots

It seems appropriate to consider autopilots first because they came first; Almer Sperry designed his autopilot in 1909, at a time when there were very few human pilots. Five years later in 1914 a Curtiss seaplane flew automatically across the river Seine, guided by Sperry's son Laurence. The autopilot used a gyroscope to detect roll and pitch and operated hydraulic servo-controls to maintain stable flight. Similar systems remained in use until the 1930s, when full electrical operation came into use. Then during the 1940s, electronic devices were introduced. In 1947 a Douglas C-54 flew from Newfoundland to England with the autopilot in charge throughout the flight including take-off and landing. Developments have continued at an accelerated pace with the introduction of increasingly powerful computers.

An autopilot may be used in all phases of flight; in climbing, in level flight and in the descent, although the final part of the approach has usually been controlled by signals from the airport, as will be described below. Automatic control has recently been used to counteract the effects of turbulence.

Instrument landing systems

The earliest system relied on quick thinking by the pilot. With some guidance from the control tower, the pilot would dive into the low fog or mist, and if, when there was some visibility, the runway was straight ahead, the plane was landed. If not, the pilot overshot, climbed, turned and tried again. This was not a very relaxing procedure, particularly if it had to be repeated more than once.

Since 1950 major airports have been required to install instrument landing systems. The arrangements are illustrated diagrammatically in Fig. 5.9. There are two radio transmitters: one (the localiser) emits in a vertical plane which runs along the centre-line of the runway, the other emits along

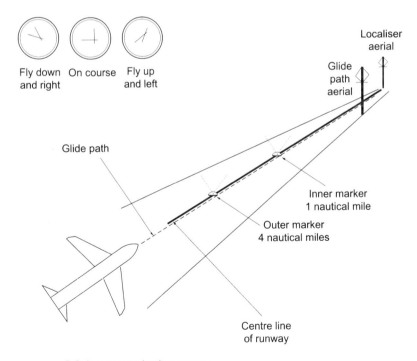

5.9 Instrument landing system.

the glide path. There are also beams that are directed vertically to show the distance from the start of the runway. The first two signals activate an instrument in the cockpit, which operates as shown in the inset to Fig. 5.9. There are two pointers; when they are respectively vertical and horizontal the aircraft has the correct heading and is flying directly down the glide path. Deviations are indicated when the pointers are in other positions, as shown.

In the approach, the pilot makes a turn which is continued until the localiser beam is picked up. The aircraft is then lined up with the beam and descends until it picks up the glide path indicator. The glide path is held until there is sufficient visibility for a manual landing. At this point the pilot decides whether or not a landing is practicable; if not, he or she overshoots.

A completely blind landing was, it is claimed, first achieved at Farnborough in 1945, during the wartime blackout. However, it was not until the 1960s that there was sufficient confidence to use such techniques on passenger-carrying flights. One of the first aircraft to operate in this way was the Vickers Trident, a three-engined short-range jet used by British European Airways. The Caravelle, a very successful French rear-engined jet, was also licensed to carry out blind landings.

Flight controls

In the early days pilots operated their control surfaces such as ailerons, rudders and flaps directly, by means of wires and rods. Later, servomotors were added to do the manual work. However, starting with Concorde and in most of the recently built large jets, movements of control levers in the cockpit are translated into electrical impulses and these in turn operate the flaps, etc. This is known as the fly-by-wire system and the wires are now being replaced by optical transmission, which is lighter. Such a system facilitates the type of computer control mentioned earlier; it is lighter than mechanical control and it is cheaper to install and maintain. On the other hand, electrical, and particularly electronic, systems are vulnerable to damage in electric storms. So Concorde, for example, had a backup control system. It is hard to see how safety can be assured without such backup.

For civil aircraft it is generally accepted that the risk of catastrophic failure must be less than 10^{-7} per hour. Since the failure probability of the more sensitive electronic or electrical systems in a fly-by-wire aircraft can be up to 10^{-4} per hour, this means that in the case of automatic flight control, for example, it is necessary to duplicate, triplicate or quadruplicate circuits. There may be a considerable weight and cost penalty for providing such multiple systems and in some cases it is possible to use detectors that are capable of finding the fault and reconfiguring the system sufficiently quickly (typically this must be done within about 0.2 s) to avoid catastrophe. The technology is sophisticated and appears to be successful; Boeing put less than 2% of total aircraft losses into the category 'instruments and electricals'.

Air traffic control

The first international agreement on the control of aircraft movements was achieved at the Versailles Peace Conference in 1919 and a high level of international co-operation is still the rule.

The first air traffic controllers were men with flags. Waving the flags cleared the aircraft for take-off. In the late 1920s and 1930s custom-built airports began to appear, one such being Croydon airport, south of London. A feature of these airports was the control tower, from which aircraft movements were co-ordinated. The first radio-equipped tower was at Cleveland Municipal Airport in 1930. In the USA the principal airlines established a control system based on Newark, Chicago and Cleveland, and in 1935 the US government took over the operation and increased the number of centres quite rapidly. In the early days control was by direct communication between tower and pilot. Aircraft were cleared for landing or take-off by verbal instruction.

A major step forward came with the installation of radar. This enabled controllers to see the aircraft on their screen, but the identity and altitude were obtained from the pilot. Then methods of identifying the aircraft and measuring its altitude were developed, such that much of the information is processed by computer and displayed on a screen. In the latest technique, installed in Europe and the USA during 1995–98, the operation is automated and clearance is given automatically by the computers. However, air traffic controllers retain the responsibility for separation of aircraft, which is 8–16 km horizontally and 300 m vertically.

After obtaining clearance for departure from the airport tower, an aircraft operating over land passes through a series of geographical sectors, each of which is individually controlled. The sector controllers clear the aircraft to enter their airspace and eventually hand the aircraft over to the neighbouring controller. These operations are guided by display screens which show the position and movement of each aircraft, as determined by radar. If at any point in the chain a controller cannot accept an aircraft, it is stacked in a holding pattern which maintains the specified vertical and horizontal separation. No system is perfect, of course, but the technological improvements in this field have greatly reduced the risk of mid-air collision.

Passenger safety

In view of the phenomenal rate at which aeronautics has progressed since the beginning of the twentieth century, it is not surprising that safety has likewise improved. Nearly all the technological change has been in a positive direction so far as safety is concerned: the rapid increase in engine power, the increased strength of the airframe due to all-metal construction, automation of controls, the development of blind landing methods and improved air traffic control have all made contributions to a reduction in fatality rates of 3.5% annually.

Shipping

The Lloyd's Register data quoted in Chapter 1 showed a steady fall in the percentage loss of shipping extending from the 1890s to the 1990s. The fatality risk for seamen has fallen in a similar way. In 1900 the annual death rate was 0.14% and by 1950 it had fallen to 0.03%, corresponding to an annual decrement of 3%. Recently casualty rates have fallen in a similar way. Such improvements have been made possible by improved technology, although legislation and the regulations of the International Maritime Organization have no doubt played some part, and more recently better rescue services have helped.

Technological change

The nineteenth century saw changes in marine technology that were more profound and far-reaching than any that had gone before. The change from sail to steam, and from wood to iron and then to steel, occurred more or less at the same time, beginning about 1820 and being more or less complete by the beginning of the twentieth century.

The American ship *Savannah* is credited with the first steamship crossing of the Atlantic in 1819. However, the *Savannah*, in common with other early vessels of its type, was really a wooden sailing vessel with an auxiliary engine driving paddle wheels. The paddle wheels could be detached and stowed on deck and this is where they stayed for all but eight hours of the 21-day voyage. In practice, most of the early steamships were packet boats, providing a regular passenger service on coastal or cross-channel routes. They carried sails which could be used to save coal in a favourable wind or when the engine broke down. The steam engines themselves were very large, with pistons having a stroke of up to 6 ft and diameters as large as 7 ft. At the time boiler shells were made of low-strength iron plates and the maximum steam pressure available was about 5 psi, so to obtain sufficient power a large-diameter cylinder was required.

Paddle steamers were not comfortable ships in high seas. It was necessary to locate the paddle shaft well above the water line so the centre of gravity of the machinery was high, consequently the ships rolled badly. When they rolled, one paddle came out of the water and the other ploughed in, causing a corkscrew motion. Nevertheless, unlike sailing ships they were independent of the wind and could maintain regular schedules with much shorter journey times. The steamer companies thus got the mail contracts and this helped to finance expensive development (as happened with aircraft nearly a hundred years later). Two lines in particular benefited in this way: Cunard, which had the main share of the transatlantic traffic and P&O (originally the Peninsular and Oriental Steam Navigation Company), which pioneered the Eastern routes, eventually to India. Figure 5.10 shows the *William Fawcett*, considered to be the first steam paddle ship operated by P&O for regular passenger and mail services. Figure 5.11 pictures one of their early screw-driven ships.

The screw propeller was invented in 1838 but it was a long time before it was universally adopted. Cunard took delivery of their first propeller-driven ship in 1862, partly because Samuel Cunard, who founded

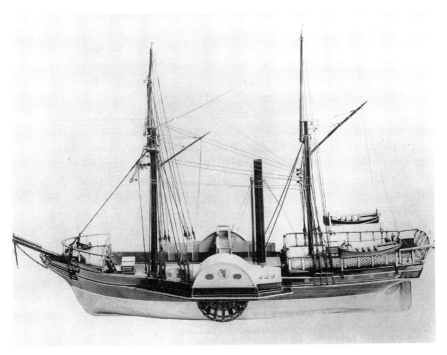

5.10 A model of the 206-ton *William Fawcett* built in 1828, intended for the P&O service between the British Isles and Spain and Portugal.

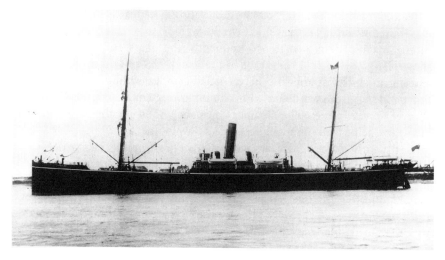

5.11 The 3174-ton *Hong Kong* propeller steamship built for P&O in 1889.

the company, thought the old ways were best. Isambard Kingdom Brunel took a different view and his *Great Britain*, launched in 1843, was the first large ship to use a propeller. It was also one of the early iron ships. Iron provided the rigidity that was necessary for the propeller and its shaft.

Not all Brunel's innovations were successful. A major disadvantage of wood as a structural material was that the greatest length of ship for which it could be used was about 300 ft. Brunel's iron ship *Great Eastern*, launched in 1859, was over twice as long with a displacement of over 18 000 tons. It was by far the largest ship afloat at the time and it was equipped with both screw propellers and paddle wheels. However, on her first crossing of the Atlantic, high seas broke off the paddle wheels and smashed the rudder. During that period Atlantic liners used to carry a cow to provide fresh milk for the passengers. Unfortunately the broken paddle demolished the cow-house and precipitated the cow through a skylight on to the passengers in the saloon below. Subsequently the *Great Eastern* failed to attract passengers and finished up laying the transatlantic telephone cable.

The first iron ships were constructed around 1840 and by 1890 very few wooden ships were being made (Fig. 5.12). Towards the end of the nineteenth century steel became cheaper than iron, so shipbuilders and designers were able to take advantage of its higher strength. Steel also enabled boiler manufacturers, who had already developed iron boilers to a considerable extent, to increase steam pressure still further. Higher pressures made compound engines possible, in which the exhaust from a small high-pressure cylinder passed to a larger low-pressure cylinder. This

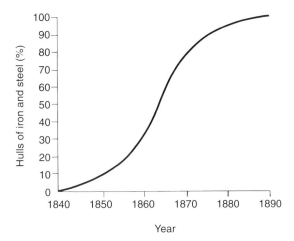

5.12 Ships built of iron and steel as a percentage of the total 1840–90.

principle was extended to triple expansion and quadruple expansion engines, which provided greater power and were more economical. The ultimate development of these reciprocating steam engines was a quadruple expansion type working with superheated steam at 400 psi, incorporating reheat.

The steam turbine was developed by the end of the nineteenth century and became the preferred type of engine for warships and large passenger ships. After the Second World War they were also used in cargo ships, container ships and tankers. Diesel engines also became competitive for ship propulsion between the world wars and have become increasingly dominant in recent years.

The first steamers had a displacement of a few hundred tons and were very small ships indeed by current standards. The size increased quite rapidly, particularly in the case of transatlantic liners, which set the pace. The first of these, the Cunard ship *Britannia*, was 207 ft long and displaced 1145 tons. She was a square-rigged wooden paddle steamer and very uncomfortable. Charles Dickens took passage to Boston on her in 1842. By the 1880s the sails had almost gone and the tonnage had gone up typically to about 7000 tons. Around this time the notion that a passenger liner could be a floating hotel began to take shape and the next generation, including two ill-fated ships the *Lusitania* and the *Titanic*, had very luxurious first-class accommodation. The *Lusitania* displaced 31 550 tons and the *Titanic* 46 383 tons. The final phase for the big transatlantic liners, before their trade was taken over by the airlines, came with the launching of the *Queen Mary* in 1934, at over 80 000 tons displacement.

Liners still operate on pleasure cruises, but they have not continued to grow in size. The *Oreana*, launched in 1995, displaces 69 153 tons.

Size is clearly an advantage in the battle against wind and weather, but it is no guarantee of safety, as the loss of the *Titanic* demonstrated. It might be thought that at least it would ensure a smooth crossing, but this too was not always the case. The Atlantic weather in 1936, the year of the *Queen Mary*'s maiden voyage from Liverpool to New York, was the worst that anyone could remember. Unfortunately the new ship rolled badly. At the height of one storm an upright piano in the tourist class lounge tore itself loose and crashed around, smashing furniture and tearing off the panelling. A number of passengers were injured and when the ship arrived in New York, to a tumultuous welcome, there was a line of ambulances waiting, parked discreetly out of sight. The problem took a year to rectify.

Cargo vessels went through a similar cycle of growth, which culminated in the construction of great supertankers, followed by stabilisation at a more modest size. One of the vital factors in the growth of the cargo fleet – numerically rather than in size – was the establishment of a network of telegraphic communications in the industrialised countries. The first successful submarine telegraph cable was laid between Britain and France in 1851 and a transatlantic link followed in 1858. This system made possible the operation of tramp ships which, having discharged a cargo, received instructions as to where next to proceed. The tramp steamer was a relatively small general-purpose ship that dominated the scene until after the Second World War, when specialised vessels started to appear. There were oil tankers already, but bulk carriers for such cargoes as iron ore and grain were developed. Then in the 1960s the container revolutionised the transit of cargo. Goods were stowed into standardised containers at warehouses remote from the ports and loaded mechanically on specially adapted ships. This eliminated the traditional dock labour and greatly reduced pilfering, which had been an ancient tradition at ports and a constant source of loss. Special ships were also made for transporting liquefied natural gas and other refrigerated cargoes.

There is no doubt that standards of both design and construction have improved substantially in the post-1945 period. Failures such as the Liberty ships and the *Sea Gem* cast a long shadow and materials have been radically improved, as described earlier. Design has, with the assistance of the computer, become more exact and sophisticated. Altogether it is becoming less and less likely that failures will occur because of gross deficiencies in material, design or construction. It is not, of course, possible to provide for the worst excesses of storm and tempest, nor is it possible to eliminate human error. But the navigational aids described below are improving progressively, in such a way as to minimise these two hazards.

Navigation

In the nineteenth century the navigation of a ship relied on three essential aids: an accurate chart, the ability to determine position and the measurement of the ship's speed together with an estimation of its drift due to wind and current. Latitude was measured by making astronomical observations with a sextant. Longitude was obtained by noting the time at which the sun had reached its zenith. Every four minutes after 12 o'clock noon represented one degree east of the Greenwich meridian, and vice versa, so that an accurate chronometer was required. Speed was obtained by throwing a plank over the stern of the ship. Attached to the plank was a cord which was knotted at regular intervals. The seaman counted the number of knots that passed through the hand during a period of 30 s; this gave the speed, in knots, naturally. Having determined latitude and longitude, the navigator was able to use the chart in order to measure the course to be set and this course was maintained by the helmsman by means of a magnetic compass.

By the year 1900 the required skills were so developed that a good navigator could, in favourable weather, determine a ship's position with reasonable accuracy. Fair weather was not always to hand, though, and the advent of wireless was a major step in resolving the remaining uncertainties.

Wireless (originally wireless telegraphy, now radio) became a practical aid to marine navigation after Marconi made the first transatlantic transmission from Cornwall to Massachusetts. Wireless quickly became standard equipment on large vessels. It enabled them to maintain contact with shore and with other vessels and to send out distress calls when necessary. Time signals were sent out daily from Greenwich, enabling navigators to correct their chronometers. In the original Marconi system, the radio signal was generated by an electric spark and comprised a spectrum of wavelengths; receivers converted these signals into an on–off electric current. Voice transmission was not possible and all communication was made using the Morse code. The practical effect, however, was dramatic and great public interest was aroused; for example when the American ship *Republic* collided with the Italian *Florida* in 1909, wireless signals from the *Republic* brought help within half an hour and the entire complement of both ships, amounting to 1700 passengers, was saved. In the same year Dr Crippen, having murdered his wife in London, was escaping with his mistress to the USA when, as a result of a wireless message, he was arrested on board ship. And then there was the *Titanic* disaster. Few, if any, technological changes have had such a startling impact as radio communication.

Following the invention of the thermionic valve in 1904 and subsequent developments in electrical circuits, the transmission of speech became possible just before the First World War. The internationally agreed distress call in speech was 'Mayday', which is an anglicisation of the French *m'aidez*.

Even before these developments, it was found possible to use a radio receiver to determine the direction from which a signal had come. Radio beacons had begun to supplement or replace lighthouses and a ship could find its position without astronomical observations and in any weather other than a severe electrical storm. The sextant was put away for good.

In about 1925 echo-sounding devices came into use, replacing the ancient lead weight and line method. In their present manifestation, echo-sounding (also known as sonar) systems are fitted below the hull of the ship and emit a series of ultrasonic pulses. Electric counters measure the time of reflection of the pulses from the sea bed and convert such measurements into distance. The result is displayed on a cathode-ray tube or a piece of paper. This aid to navigation was used to detect submarines during the First World War.

During the 1930s the possibility of using radio waves for echo location began to be explored, particularly in Britain, Germany and the USA. The Germans had produced such a device in 1933, but they used too long a wavelength and the equipment was not very effective. In fact, useful results could only be obtained with a high-frequency beacon operating in the range 300–3000 megahertz. The beam is generated by a device called a magnetron and is fed to a rotating parabolic transmitter. Reflections are picked up by an antenna and the results displayed on a circular cathode-ray screen. Solid objects appear as a bright spot. Their distance from the centre of the screen represents the range and the angular displacement from the vertical is the bearing. The main incentive for this development was the need to detect aircraft during the Second World War, but its value for the avoidance of collisions at sea will be obvious. Radar is now standard equipment for most seagoing vessels Computer technology and satellite communication have further improved the navigability of ships in more recent years.

All in all, radio has conferred tremendous benefits to shipping and must have been a major factor in the improvement of safety that we have seen during the twentieth century. However, many of the other improvements that have been described here have also made a contribution and there is little doubt that the future will see yet further improvements in marine safety.

The oil and gas industry

Drilling operations

The percussion method has been used for drilling deep wells by the Chinese for over a thousand years and came into use in Western Europe and America towards the end of the eighteenth century. This technique employed a metal bit shaped like a chisel to break up rock and bore through it. The tool was alternately raised and then allowed to drop; for example in the Chinese method the bit was suspended by a rope from one end of a plank which pivoted like a see-saw and the drillers took turns to jump on the end of the plank, so giving the tool a reciprocating motion.

Percussion drilling was used mainly to extract salt, which often occurs as 'salt domes' lying below a cap of rock. When Colonel Drake drilled the first oil well in Pennsylvania in 1859 he employed a salt driller to do the work. By this time the steam engine had been harnessed to provide the up-and-down motion, as shown in Fig. 5.13. The tool was now suspended on a wire rope and a derrick provided the means to hoist the bit and other devices into and out of the well. The system became known as cable-tool drilling.

The rotating cutter rockbit was invented by Howard Hughes and came into use during the first decade of the twentieth century. This tool became more generally used in subsequent years but cable-tool drilling continued

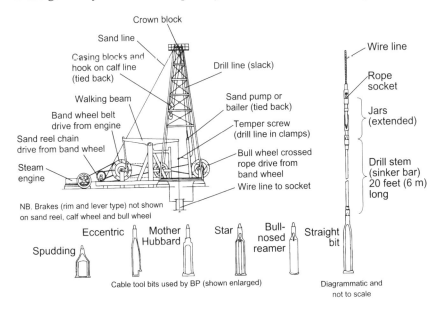

5.13 Cable-tool drilling rig.

to dominate the scene. Then the financial crisis of 1930 halted oil drilling completely for two years. When operations resumed, the competitive climate favoured rotary drilling and the cable tool fell out of use.

Rotary drilling introduced a radically new method of removing the spoil. Previously this had been taken out periodically by a bailer, which was essentially a tubular can with a self-closing bottom. In rotary drilling a circulating fluid was employed which flushed out the ground rock and conveyed it to the surface. In making a vertical hole, the drill is rotated by a tubular shaft known as the string. A liquid flows down inside the string and then up through the annular space between the string and the well casing. As well as carrying away spoil, this fluid (called mud) cools the drill head and provides a hydrostatic head which helps to counter the pressure in the oil-bearing formation (down-hole pressure). The mud is circulated from a tank down and up the well, then over a shaker which separates the chippings, and back to the mud tank (Fig. 5.14).

Oil wells go very deep and the pressure is correspondingly very high. It is normal practice to fit a non-return valve in the string just above the drill head to prevent an uncontrolled upward flow. However, accidents may happen; the string may fracture or come unscrewed, or the drill may break unexpectedly into a high-pressure region. Therefore the well-head is fitted with means of countering such emergencies. Figure 5.15 illustrates a blowout preventer of the type commonly fitted to land-based wells and some offshore wells. The top preventer has a large rubber element capable of sealing around any tool or around the drill string. The middle ram will close the annular space around the string, while the lower, blind ram consists of two flat-faced elements that meet in the centre and seal off the well completely. If a drill string is present, the tube is crushed. These closures may be individually and separately operated by the drilling crew according to the prevailing emergency. In less pressing circumstances an excess in down-hole pressure may be countered by increasing the density of the mud. This is usually accomplished by the addition of barytes (barium sulphate).

Oilfield development

There are three main stages in the establishment and exploitation of an oil or gas field. The first step is to carry out a seismic survey to identify rock structures that could be oil bearing. Offshore, this was at first done by detonating a propane–oxygen mixture in a rubber container and analysing the reflections from the sub-sea strata. An alternative source is a high-energy vibrator. Explosives are no longer used because of the damage caused to marine life.

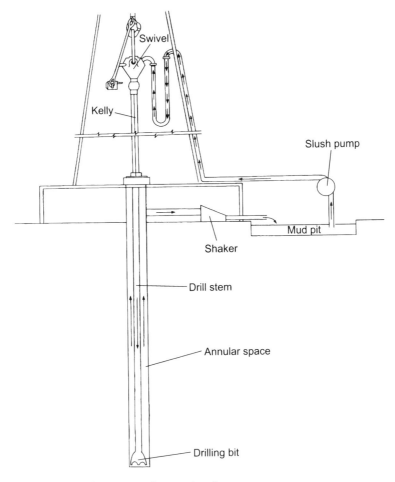

5.14 The mud flow system for an oil well.

When a likely area is found its boundaries are determined and then an exploratory vertical well is drilled somewhere close to the centre. This is the wildcat well and is generally considered to be the most hazardous of the drilling operations, because the composition and pressure of any hydrocarbon that may be present is unknown. If results from the first well are positive, other exploratory wells are drilled with the object of defining the extent of the field.

In the third phase an offshore field is developed by establishing fixed platforms and using these as a base to drill production wells. Sometimes there will be only a single vertical well; more often multiple wells are sunk.

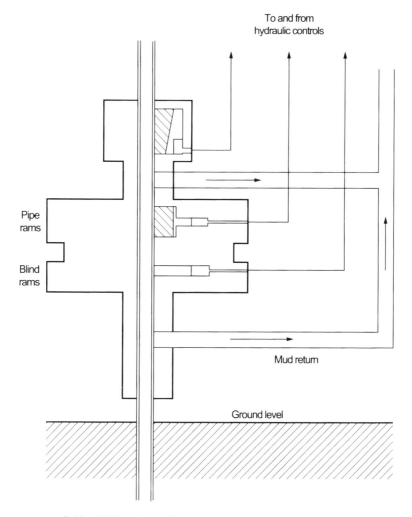

5.15 Well head with blowout preventer: sectional diagram.

In order to cover the area assigned to the platform, wells must be dug at an angle to the vertical (directional wells: Fig. 5.16). To do this, turbodrills are used. These drills are driven by a water turbine mounted behind the head. The turbine itself is driven by mud flow down the string. Using this device it is possible to drill wells at angles of up to 45° from vertical. As these are completed the wells are tied in to the separation unit and then via an export riser to the sub-sea pipeline that takes the product onshore.

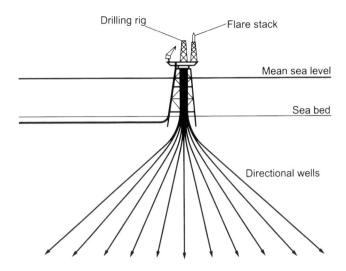

5.16 Development drilling from a fixed offshore platform.

Blowouts

Blowouts are a particular hazard offshore because not only are they a danger to life and limb but, in the case of any oil blowout, they also generate an oil slick and much unfavourable publicity. The majority of blowouts, however, result from the sudden release of gas.

Figures gathered by the US Geological Survey indicate that for the period 1953–71 blowouts occurred in 0.02% of the wells that were drilled and that this rate did not vary significantly.[3] A later report from the Minerals Management Service of the US Department of the Interior covering the period 1971–85 also indicated no significant change in the blowout rate. The WOAD data for 1970 to 1987 shows that blowout accidents that resulted in fatalities did not vary significantly. About one-third of the incidents related to fixed units (jackets) and presumably took place when drilling development wells. The risk is evidently not confined to exploratory drilling. WOAD data indicate that if supercatastrophes are excluded, blowout accounts for 36% of all fatalities on fixed units, compared with 13% on mobile units.

Blowouts are an intractable problem. It would appear that blowout protectors, if properly maintained and operated by skilled people, are reliable and capable of controlling a well in an emergency. However, a rapid build-up of pressure or loss of circulating fluid, or simple human error can all lead to loss of control and it is difficult to see how technological progress can have very much effect on this situation.

The development of offshore structures

The drilling of underwater oil wells started during the 1920s in Louisiana and in Lake Maracaibo, Venezuela. Piles were driven into the lake bed and these supported a relatively small structure and platform, on which were mounted the derrick and power units. Ancillary equipment was carried on a tender moored alongside. When the well was completed the derrick was removed, leaving the platform with its production well-head. A similar type of operation was conducted from jetties or piers off the Californian coast.

Increasing demand for oil and gas after the Second World War forced operating companies to consider extending their activities to the continental shelf. In 1945 President Truman signed a proclamation laying claim to all the mineral rights in the regions off the coast of the United States. This claim was confirmed by the Geneva Convention on the Continental Shelf in 1958. Meantime there has been continued development of offshore technology. In the 1940s the first self-contained offshore units were built. These were flat-bottomed barges which were towed out to the required position. By flooding buoyancy compartments they were made to settle on the sea bed with the drilling platform above the waterline. Such operations were mainly confined to shallow water in the Mexican Gulf.

Platforms of this type are designated 'submersibles'. In recent years sub-sea vehicles or submarines have also been categorised as 'submersibles', so there is scope for confusion. So far as this book is concerned submarines are submarines and submersibles are the type of offshore platform referred to above.

In the 1950s, to cope with the requirement for drilling at greater depths, submersibles were further developed by building the platform on columns supported by a submerged flooded pontoon. Such units have operated in up to 175 ft of water. Jack-up platforms appeared during the same period. These, as we have seen in the case of the *Sea Gem*, were adaptations of self-elevating platforms used for general engineering purposes. In the late 1950s two types of floating platform appeared: the semi-submersibles and the drill ship. Semi-submersibles, which float on submerged pontoons, are held in position by a system of anchors generally similar to that described for the *Alexander L Kielland* and can drill to depths of 1500 ft. The drill ship, which can drill down to 6000 ft or more, appeared at about the same time. At first, this was an adapted merchant vessel, moored like a semi-submersible, but in the 1960s purpose-built vessels with dynamic positioning equipment were introduced. Figure 5.17 illustrates these developments.

Submersibles, semi-submersibles, jack-up platforms and drill ships are all mobile units and are normally used for drilling exploration wells.

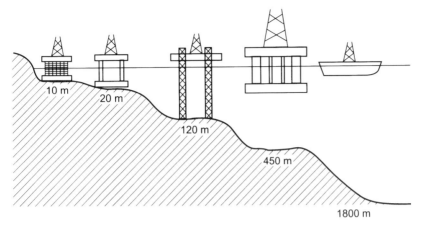

5.17 Development of offshore drilling rigs.

Development wells are drilled from fixed units, which may also carry primary separation equipment and gas or oil exporting pipelines. There are four main types: jackets, artificial islands, concrete structures and tension leg platforms. Jackets have been described elsewhere; *Piper Alpha* was typical of such platforms. Artificial islands are exactly what the name suggests. They are made by dredging sand or gravel from nearby and dumping it to make an island, from which drilling operations can be conducted more or less as on dry land. Artificial islands may have an advantage in shallow arctic waters where structures could be damaged by ice. Reinforced concrete is used for very large bases that rest by gravity on the sea bed. A platform of normal metal construction is mounted on top of the concrete columns. Tension leg platforms resemble jackets, but are mounted on pontoons, like a semi-submersible, to give positive buoyancy. The whole system is tethered to the sea bed by tension members. Tension leg platforms are intended for operating in waters that are too deep (over about 800 ft) for a conventional jacket and are coming into use as a means of extending operations into deeper waters. Figure 5.18 shows the Conoco Hutton tension leg platform which operated in the North Sea.

The record is one of rapid technological change, in which completely new types of drilling platform have been developed. It is not surprising in these circumstances that the fatality rate has been high. During the period 1970–87 nearly 60% of the casualties occurred as the result of four major losses of mobile units. One of these, the *Alexander L Kielland*, was of a type that is unlikely to recur. The others were sunk in heavy seas and whilst this risk will always remain, improved stability and better evacuation procedures could greatly reduce the fatality rates. One of the negative

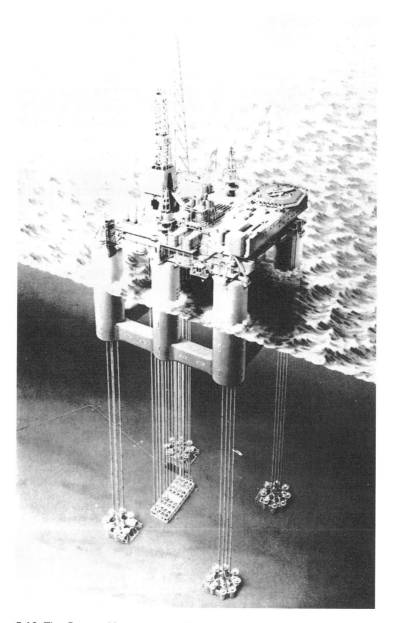

5.18 The Conoco Hutton tension leg platform.

factors in the case of offshore operations is that the improvements in navigation and guidance systems that have had such a beneficial effect for aircraft and for normal shipping do not make much difference to the safety of mobile drilling units. Moreover, improvements in safety are to some degree countered by the need to operate at increasing depths. Nevertheless, experience in the 1980s had led to some useful developments. The very radical changes in the layout of jackets following the *Piper Alpha* disaster are described in Chapter 3; these represent a substantial contribution to safety. After the *Alexander L Kielland* accident and the capsizing of *Ocean Ranger* in 1982, the classification societies required that redundancy should be incorporated in the structure and that the platform should be capable of floating. Some of the more recent semi-submersibles have accommodated these requirements by using twin floaters (pontoons) on which are mounted braced rectangular columns supporting the platform.

Hydrocarbon processing

In 1784 Ami Argand, a Swiss distiller, invented a new type of oil lamp, which was to usher in great improvements in domestic comfort. In earlier times oil lamps produced a deal of smoke and smell, but very little light. Argand used a circular wick around which was mounted a glass chimney, such that air was drawn up on either side of the wick. This produced a bright clear flame, giving a light equal to 10 or 12 tallow candles. The same principle is used in oil lamps to this day. Unfortunately for Argand, his partner allowed the patent to lapse and within a year or two the design had been pirated and 'Argand Patent Lamps' were on sale in London.

Gas lighting and the means of producing illuminating gas from coal were developed in the 1790s by William Murdock and by 1802 had been used to light a factory in Birmingham. The streets of Baltimore were lit by coal gas as early as 1816. Domestic use developed more slowly, partly because of the need for a piped supply system, and was restricted to towns. In country areas (and in the nineteenth century a high proportion of the population lived in the country) illumination was, other than in a few big houses, by candles and oil lamps.

The oil used for the Argand lamp and its subsequent developments was rape oil (then known as colza oil) or alternatively whale oil. These liquids were too viscous to be drawn up by a wick, so various ingenious means were used to bring the oil close to the flame. In the Argand and other lamps it was fed by gravity and in others by mechanical devices. Kerosene, known in Britain as paraffin, is non-viscous and can readily be drawn up a cotton wick. In the 1840s and 1850s it was obtained by distillation from coal and from oil shale. So when Colonel Drake struck oil in Pennsylvania in 1859 there was a large established market for lamp oil. It may be argued, therefore, that Ami Argand was the true father of the oil industry.

Initially, kerosene was the only marketable product to be obtained from crude oil; the remainder was discarded or burnt. However, during the last quarter of the nineteenth and first half of the twentieth century the gas industry found it expedient to supplement supplies of coal gas with semi-watergas, which is made by passing a mixture of air and steam through red-hot coke. This produces a mixture of hydrogen, carbon monoxide and nitrogen which burns well but has a lower calorific value than coal gas. To make up the difference, gas oil, which is the next higher boiling fraction of crude oil after kerosene, was injected into the gas via a carburettor. The carburettor worked in the same way as that of a petrol engine by spraying a fine jet of hydrocarbon into a gas stream, thereby vaporising and mixing it with the gas. The product was known as carburetted water gas.

Then at the end of the nineteenth century the internal combustion engine was invented. Petrol engines were fuelled by gasoline, a lighter fraction than kerosene and diesel engines by diesel oil, which is the same as gas oil. Vehicles were (and are) fuelled by light diesel, or light gas oil, and marine engines by heavy diesel, or heavy gas oil.

The term 'fraction' comes from the fractional distillation process, which is the basic petroleum refinery operation. Distillation is carried out in a tower in which the vapour flow is from bottom to top and the temperature is highest at the bottom (Figs 5.19 and 5.20). The tower contains trays on which products that condense over a specific temperature range collect and these are drained off, usually for further treatment. Table 5.2 shows approximate boiling ranges for the different fractions available from a typical crude oil. It must be remembered, however, that the composition of crude oil varies greatly from place to place, so this tabulation is not universally applicable.

So in the early twentieth century the oil industry changed from being a supplier of illuminating oil and gas to being a supplier of power.[4] All fractions were now used. The residual oil eventually replaced coal as a fuel for steam boilers on ships. As the use of motor cars increased, so did the demand for gasoline and means were found (thermal and later catalytic cracking) to break down the heavier molecules and increase the gasoline yields. Refineries grew larger and crude oil was increasingly transported (in the USA) by pipeline.

Pipelines were an early example of the use of welding for pressurised equipment. The individual pipe lengths were made by forming plate to shape and then making a longitudinal weld in a very large flash butt-welding machine. After removing the flash from the weld, the pipes were stretched by means of a hydraulically operated internal mandrel. This

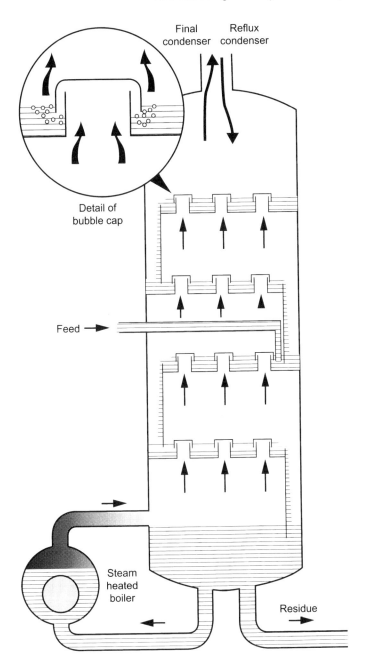

Final condenser   Reflux condenser

Detail of bubble cap

Feed →

Steam heated boiler

Residue →

5.19 Distillation (bubble) tower: vapour rising through the tower bubbles through the liquid held on successive trays, stripping out the lighter fractions which are taken towards the top.

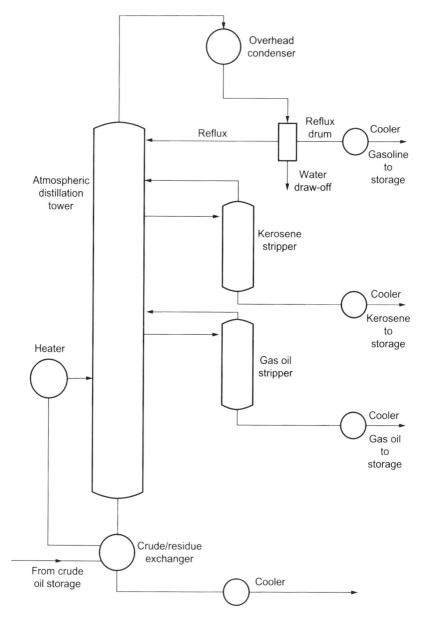

5.20 Crude oil distillation.

Table 5.2 Approximate boiling ranges

Fraction or product	Boiling range (°C)
Gasoline	65–90
Benzene	90–140
Naphtha	140–165
Kerosene	165–240
Light gas oil (light diesel)	240–320
Heavy gas oil (heavy diesel)	320–365
Residue	over 365

operation tested the weld and at the same time increased the yield strength. Then in the field, the pipes were welded end-to-end by a manual technique known as stovepipe welding, using electrodes that consisted of wire wrapped with paper sealed with sodium silicate. The field welds were porous but this problem was overcome by wrapping with oil-soaked ropes or by encasing in concrete. The pipelining technique so developed has lasted almost unchanged to the present day, except that the field welds are no longer porous.

Otherwise, refineries were of riveted construction. A big change took place, however, after the Second World War. Fusion welding was introduced as a means of fabricating most items of refinery equipment, together with the interconnecting pipework. The oil industry played a major part in improving welding methods and inspection techniques, and wrote codes for the construction of pressure vessels and pipework. As a result, it became possible to use fabricated process plants for high-pressure operations on a large scale.

High-pressure technology had been developed early in the twentieth century primarily as a result of the invention of the Haber–Bosch process for synthesising ammonia. In this process, a mixture of hydrogen and nitrogen was passed over an iron catalyst at a pressure of up to 200 atm. In order to contain such pressure, it was necessary to use large forgings and although forged ammonia converters of up to 300 tons in weight were eventually produced, this requirement was a serious limitation.

In the post-1945 years, the techniques that had been developed for hydrocarbon processing were applied to a modified form of the Haber process which operated at a somewhat lower pressure. The final result was a single-train plant using a centrifugal compressor capable of producing 1000 tons or more of ammonia per day, which was much higher than was possible with the old Haber–Bosch process. The new process also provided a route to the production of nitric acid. Thus, hydrocarbon processing technology has now provided the most economic means of fixing nitrogen, which was the traditional activity of the heavy inorganic chemical industry.

Hydrocracking is another technique requiring high pressure. This process is used to break down the heaviest of crude oil fractions, including residual oils, to form lighter and potentially more marketable products. The hydrogenation is carried out at a pressure of about 2000 psi in stainless-clad heavy-wall reactors.

One of the major developments of post-1945 years has been the growth of the plastics industry. One of the raw materials for this industry is ethylene, which is produced by the pyrolysis of methane at a relatively low pressure. Low-density polyethylene (of the sort used for polythene bags, for example) is produced at high pressure in a reactor made of forged alloy steel.

Alongside these process changes, the technique of fabricating process plants has improved steadily; steels are less subject to embrittlement and welding techniques are more reliable. The failure of welded joints has not at any time been a serious problem in process plant operation, so these improvements have not significantly affected safety in hydrocarbon processing.

Land transport

The movement of goods and individuals within Britain, continental Europe and the United States is by air, rail, road and by waterways. Air transport has already been discussed, whilst of the other three, railways and roads provide the main hazards so far as human fatalities and injuries are concerned.

The nineteenth century saw a major development of railway systems, whilst roads were relatively neglected. In the twentieth century, by contrast, road transport has become predominant. The numbers of rail passengers increased up to the First World War, then remained more or less consistent until the last decade or so, when there has been a modest increase. Overall, the result has been a great increase in both speed and range of movements of all kinds. The total number of casualties has not, however, risen in proportion; on the contrary, as the figures quoted in Chapter 2 demonstrate, they have either remained constant or have fallen, whilst the accident rate has been reduced, in some cases (road traffic accidents for example) quite dramatically.

Railways

Rail casualties fall into one of four categories: those due to the movement of trains, those occurring in train accidents, level crossing accidents, or suicide and trespass. The effect of technological change is most pronounced in the case of train accidents. Casualties from such events decrease with the passage of time, but the record may be distorted periodically by catastrophes such as that at Eschede.

One of the most important developments in passenger rolling stock was the construction of carriages made from steel instead of wood. One of the most potentially lethal effects of a rail crash is that carriages tend to override the one in front. Steel vehicles are much more likely to survive such events intact than those made of wood. Developments along these lines continue, with the progressive strengthening of carriages. Improvements in braking also contribute to safety. With early air or vacuum brakes those at the rear of a long train came on several seconds after those at the front. Development of electro-vacuum systems during the inter-war years eliminated this problem.

The most important means of avoiding train accidents is the system used for controlling rail movements. An essential element of such a system is the signal that warns train drivers to proceed cautiously or to stop. Originally this was a semaphore-type indicator operated by levers and rods. This was replaced by electric light devices, which were later augmented by audio signals in the driver's cab. Some railways also arranged for automatic application of the brakes at a stop signal. A final step (short of completely automatic operation) is to dispense with trackside instruments altogether and rely on the audio signals. This system has been adopted successfully on at least one freight line in the USA.

Heavier trains and increased speeds made it necessary to improve the quality of the track. Wooden sleepers were replaced by concrete or steel ones. Rails are welded end-to-end in order to provide a smoother and quieter ride for passengers. More important from a safety viewpoint was the track circuit. This system, invented in 1872 but not adopted until the beginning of the twentieth century, enabled the position of trains to be displayed in signal boxes. More recently, the use of computers has made such techniques progressively more sophisticated. They do not, however, have the ability to make the trains run on time.

Road transport

In general, developments in road transport have proceeded along two main lines: improvements in the reliability and safety of vehicles and the construction and maintenance of a better road network.

Reference 1 of Chapter 2 shows that per mile, motorways are the safest type of road, so they may be credited with a contribution to safety, as well as providing for the rapid transit of goods and services. The proper marking of lanes on all types of road is an important means of guiding drivers and maintaining driving discipline. Control at intersections by traffic signals and roundabouts minimises the risk of side impact collisions. It is difficult to judge the relative value of such measures. Relevant information on the causes of road traffic accidents is not generally available.

During the last quarter of the twentieth century the reliability of motor vehicles improved greatly, in part through the use of electronic controls, but also because of a general improvement in braking systems, power units and transmission. Reliability is important in road transport because breakdowns can result in a serious disruption of traffic flow and this in turn may increase the risk of accidents.

Much work has been done to improve the strength of the car body and to turn it into a protective capsule. The discipline of crashworthiness has also made good contributions to car safety. An important aspect of this work is the measurement of the amount of energy that is absorbed by the vehicle body when a collision occurs. The greater the amount of energy absorption, the lower the risk of injury to the passengers. Crashworthiness techniques are applicable to all forms of transport.

References

1. Wallner, F. 'The LD process', *Metal Construction*, 1986 **8** 28–33.
2. Middleton, D. *Civil Aviation, a Design History*, Ian Allan, Shepperton, 1986.
3. Lowson, M.H. (ed), *Our Industry – Petroleum*, British Petroleum, London, 1970.
4. Williams, T.I. *A Short History of Twentieth Century Technology*, Clarendon Press, Oxford, 1982.

CHAPTER 6

Natural catastrophes

Natural catastrophes and a country's level of productivity

This book is concerned primarily with those accidents that befall human artefacts such as ships, aircraft, process plant or other industrial structures. It is nevertheless relevant to consider those disasters that are caused primarily by natural forces such as hurricanes, floods and earthquakes.

There are two main reasons for so doing. In the first place, it is necessary to establish the relative scale of these two types of event. As will be enumerated shortly, natural disasters are several orders of magnitude more severe than engineering failures in their effects, in terms of both human and financial loss. The main efforts of those responsible for mitigating disasters should be directed accordingly.

The second reason is that engineering plays a major part in limiting the effects of natural forces. It was noted in Chapter 4 that in the 1995 earthquake that severely damaged the city of Kobe, Japan, most casualties resulted from the collapse of buildings of moderate height and that no building higher than seven storeys collapsed. Taller buildings had been constructed to codes that made allowance for seismic shock. Such earthquake-resistant buildings have demonstrated that well-engineered structures can withstand the most severe natural forces. Likewise, a combination of adequate flood defence systems with timely evacuation (in the Netherlands and in the Mississippi Valley, USA for example) has reduced the risk to human life from flooding almost to zero. Unfortunately, in many parts of the world where these and other natural hazards exist, the resources and capability to combat them are not available and their effects are increasingly severe.

On such grounds it would be expected that the human effect of natural disasters in individual countries might be inversely related to their productivity. Figure 6.1 shows that this is indeed the case. Here the number of people (a) killed and (b) affected by natural disasters per million of the population is plotted against the national output per head for those countries where a similar comparison was made for the mortality rate in

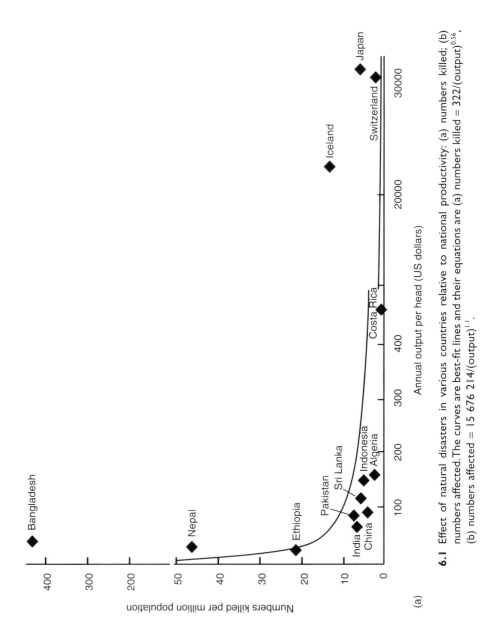

6.1 Effect of natural disasters in various countries relative to national productivity: (a) numbers killed; (b) numbers affected. The curves are best-fit lines and their equations are (a) numbers killed $= 322/(\text{output})^{0.56}$, (b) numbers affected $= 15\ 676\ 214/(\text{output})^{1.1}$.

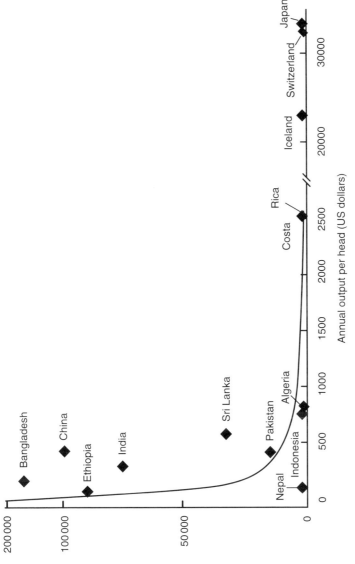

6.1 *Continued*

(b)

road accidents in Chapter 1 (Fig. 1.4). Where data are lacking, a country having similar productivity has been substituted. There is indeed an inverse relationship and in the case of numbers killed by natural disasters the various countries occupy very similar relative positions. The common factor between death from a natural disaster and death in a road accident is, of course, the fatality risk. It is implied that in any given country there is an accepted level of risk of accidental death, regardless of cause. This is an easy deduction to make; it is not so easy to explain how the level of risk may be sensed or controlled collectively by the nation as a whole.

In this chapter it is proposed to detail the incidence of natural disasters and, as an example of how engineering can combat them, to describe the evolution of earthquake-resistant building techniques in California and Japan.

The effects of natural disasters

A major source of statistical information on this subject is the *World Disasters Report*, which is published by the Oxford University Press annually for the International Federation of Red Cross and Red Crescent Societies.[1] This report also covers refugees, war and other conflicts and famines.

Data on natural disasters are maintained by the Centre for Research on the Epidemiology of Disasters, which is located at the Catholic University of Louvain, Belgium. The reported figures are annual averages of (for example) deaths, worldwide, for five successive five-year periods, whilst the database itself goes back to the year 1900.

Figure 6.2 shows the annual average number of persons killed by all types of natural disasters during the period 1972–96. The plot shows an apparent downward trend, but the correlation coefficient is too low for this trend to be statistically significant. In general, figures for deaths caused by natural disasters scatter widely and cannot be used reliably to indicate any tendency to increase or decrease with time.

The number of persons affected by disasters provides a more useful indicator, as will be seen in Fig. 6.3. There was a drop in the number of affected persons from the penultimate to the final figure. Even so, an upward trend is indicated, with a high correlation coefficient and an annual increment of 5.5%. As will be seen later, such a rise is consistent with those obtained using other criteria.

The report also includes data on 'technological accidents'. It appears reasonable to assume that this term covers events similar to those described earlier in this book. Figures for the number of persons affected by such accidents are shown in logarithmic form in Fig. 6.4, where they are compared with those for natural disasters. Natural disasters affect about a

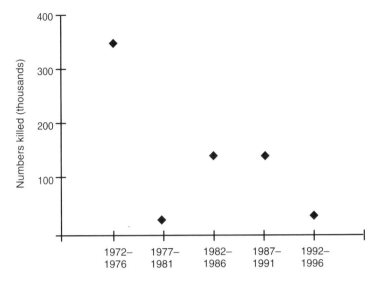

6.2 Annual average number of persons killed in natural disasters worldwide, 1972–96.

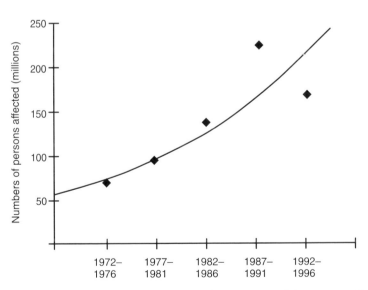

6.3 Annual average number of persons affected by natural disasters worldwide, 1972–96. Annual increment 5.5%.

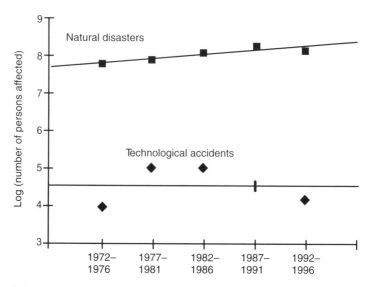

6.4 Logarithm to base 10 of the annual average number of persons affected by natural disasters and by technological accidents.

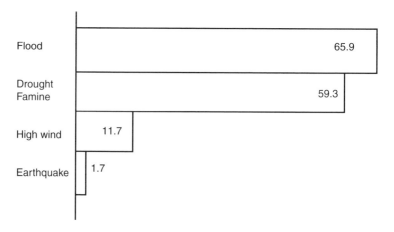

6.5 Annual average number of persons (millions) affected by natural disasters during the period 1972–96, by type of disaster.

thousand times as many people as do engineering catastrophes and much remains to be done in mitigating these numbers.

The relative effects of different types of natural event (again, in numbers of affected persons) is shown in Fig. 6.5. Flood, drought and tropical storm (high wind) predominate, whilst earthquakes, rather surprisingly, account for only about 1% of the total.

Incidence and economic effects

In May 1994 the United Nations organised a conference on natural disaster reduction in Yokohama, Japan. The incentive for this activity was made clear in the proceedings of the conference,[2] namely, that the cost of such disasters is increasing and this is having a damaging effect on the economies of some member states. For example, in the 1976 earthquake in Guatemala 24 000 people were killed and damage of US$1.1 billion was done. This cost amounted to 18% of the country's annual national income. Such international relief as may be available is never sufficient to counteract the effect of such a catastrophe.

One positive result of this conference was a study that gave figures for the effects of disasters over a 30-year period (1963–92).[2] These disasters were recorded where they produced one of the following effects:

1   Damage costing more than 1% of the annual gross national product.
2   More than 1% of the total population significantly affected.
3   Deaths of 100 or more caused.

Figure 6.6 shows the annual average number of disasters for successive five-year periods according to these criteria. All show an increasing trend, with annual increments ranging from 3.5% to 6.7%. These results are strikingly similar to those presented in the previous section, despite the different form in which the information is set out. The data source is not

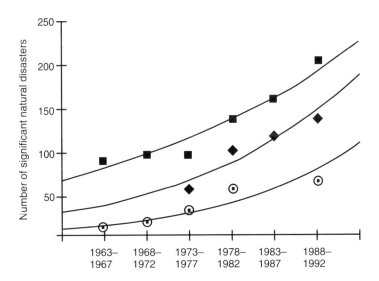

6.6 Average annual number of significant natural disasters according to the specified criteria for the period 1963–92.[2] Annual increments: significant damage (◉), 6.7%; persons affected (◆), 5.3%; deaths (■), 3.5%.

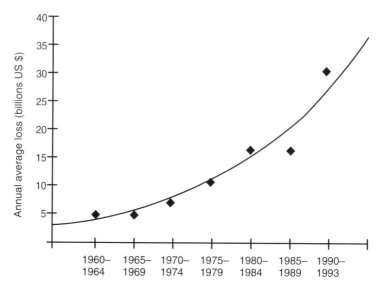

6.7 Annual average financial loss due to major natural disasters 1960–93, in billions of US dollars.[2] Annual increment 6.2%.

stated and could be the same as for the Red Cross/Red Crescent Report, since the work at Louvain University is also supported by the United Nations. However, the Yokohama Conference Report also includes data on insured and uninsured costs of natural disasters and these figures are from a different source (Munich Reinsurance). Uninsured costs are shown in Fig. 6.7, which indicates a trend very similar to disaster numbers. Note that losses resulting from natural events are measured in billions of dollars, whereas those associated with mechanical failure in process plant (Chapter 2) are in units of a million dollars, three orders of magnitude lower.

Figure 6.8 is a bar chart of the numbers of natural disasters affecting 1% or more of the population for the period 1963–92, classified according to type. The result is very similar to that for numbers of persons affected (Fig. 6.5); flood, famine and high wind are the most damaging types of event, whilst earthquakes were responsible for about 4% of the total number of disasters.

Causes

There must always be an element of doubt about data on natural catastrophes because some of the figures are produced by governments that may benefit from inflating them. Nevertheless, the material quoted above has been assembled by responsible, independent agencies and, moreover, shows a high degree of consistency. There is, therefore, little reason to doubt

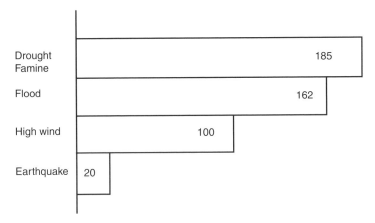

6.8 Number of natural disasters affecting 1% or more of the population during the period 1963–92, by type of disaster.

that the human effect and cost of natural disasters is increasing and that the annual rate of increase is somewhere in the region of 5%.

Three factors would appear to be responsible for this increase. The first factor is the general rise in world population, which occurs at a rate of about 2% annually. Secondly, an increasing proportion of the world's population is moving from the countryside into cities and it is urban populations that are most vulnerable to flood, high wind and earthquakes. This movement takes place also at a rate of about 2% per annum. Thirdly, both population growth and urbanisation affect primarily the less-developed regions, where the defences against natural disaster are least effective.

Earthquakes

To be involved in an earthquake is a grievous misfortune, not least because they are the most unpredictable of natural phenomena. For many years engineers and seismologists have tried to find a way of predicting the time and place of an earthquake and occasionally there is an announcement of imminent success. But nothing materialises and when the next quake occurs everyone is taken by surprise. The effects of an earthquake are equally unpredictable. There is no correlation between the energy of the event, as measured on the Richter scale, and the amount of destruction or loss of life. In part, of course, this is because many earthquakes occur in rural areas. But even when they take place in or near towns, their effects are variable.

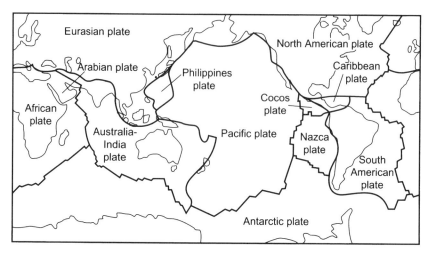

6.9 Boundaries of tectonic plates.[3]

The mechanics of the process

According to the theory of plate tectonics the Earth's crust is divided into a number of rigid plates which move relative to each other at rates of 10–100 mm per annum. Figure 6.9 shows where these plates are thought to be located.[3] At their margins the plates interact in various ways. They may slide laterally against each other, or they may collide, such that one plate rides over the other. Such movement occurs along fault lines or cracks; however, it is not a steady motion and often the crust on either side of a fault locks together until stresses build up and there is a sudden fracture. The result is a large release of energy. Elastic waves spread outwards from the fractured region, which is known as the focus. The most damaging earthquakes are caused by those where the focus is between 3 and 9 miles below the surface; these are known as shallow-focus earthquakes. Most seismic events in California are of this type, as exemplified by the 1994 earthquake at Northridge (see Fig. 6.10). The very destructive 1995 earthquake in Kobe, Japan was similar.

The theory of plate tectonics provides a good explanation of the earth movements around the Pacific ocean, notably in California and Japan. Others, however, have occurred remote from known faults or plate margins. There was a severe earthquake in 1811 which was located in the Mississippi valley. And there was once an earthquake in Birmingham, England, which caused little damage but much alarm among the local population.

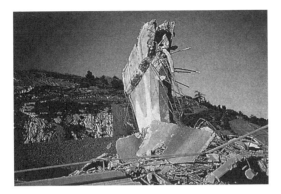

6.10 A reinforced concrete bridge span that collapsed due to the 1994 earthquake at Northridge, California.

Seismic waves

When a sudden fracture occurs, three types of elastic wave are generated: pressure or compression waves, shear waves and surface waves. Pressure waves result from horizontal movement and, at any one point, cause a fluctuating pressure; they cause little surface movement. Shear waves, on the other hand, result in violent up-and-down and side-to-side motion; these are the waves that cause most of the damage. Surface waves mainly affect the ground surface only; they may also cause both lateral and vertical movement. Pressure waves travel faster than shear waves. Thus, a seismograph will initially show a vibration of relatively small amplitude, but when the shear wave arrives the amplitude increases suddenly. The time interval between these two events provides a measure of the distance between the observation point and the epicentre of the disturbance. The epicentre is the point on the Earth's surface directly above the focus and if there are observations from two or more stations its location can be obtained.

The magnitude of an earthquake is measured using a scale proposed by the American seismologist Charles Richter in 1935. This number is the logarithm to base 10 of the maximum wave amplitude measured on a standard seismograph situated 100 km from the epicentre. The amplitude is expressed in thousandths of a millimetre. Thus, with an amplitude of one millimetre, the magnitude on the Richter scale would be 3. This number gives an estimate of the total energy of the event.

In the United States and in some other countries earthquake effects are also rated on the modified Mercalli intensity scale. This rating is subjective and is based on personal reactions to the event, amount of damage to structures and on observations of other physical effects. The intensity is indicated by a Roman numeral, with a maximum of XII.

A more important measurement, so far as destructive effect is concerned, is the acceleration of the ground surface. In principle, this figure could be obtained by analysing the seismographic record to obtain the maximum combination of amplitude and frequency. Suppose the vibration took the form of a sine wave. The maximum acceleration then occurs at the point of maximum amplitude, and is $\delta\omega^2$, where δ is amplitude and ω is frequency. In practice accelerations are best measured on the ground. The acceleration in an earthquake is usually expressed as a multiple of gravitational acceleration, g, which is $32.2\,\text{ft/s}^2$ or $9.81\,\text{m/s}^2$. Thus an acceleration of $16.1\,\text{ft/s}^2$ is expressed as $0.5\,g$. The highest accelerations so far recorded in California were during the 1994 Northridge earthquake, these being, as noted earlier, $1.8\,g$ horizontally and $1.12\,g$ vertically. A previous maximum had been $1.25\,g$ in San Fernando about 2 miles from the epicentre. Building regulations in Los Angeles require the installation of at least three accelerometers in all new multistorey buildings, so that the urban areas are well covered by these devices.

The other important factor affecting earthquake damage is the duration of the disturbance. The longer the duration, the greater the amount of damage.

The force F on the foundations of a rigid building of mass M during an earthquake causing a ground acceleration a is given by Newton's second law

$$F = Ma = MCg \qquad\qquad [6.1]$$

where C is the multiplication factor mentioned above. This quantity is known as the seismic coefficient and is much used in design for earthquake resistance.

Tidal waves

A sub-sea earthquake in which there is a large vertical displacement can produce very large waves capable of travelling considerable distances. Of course they have nothing to do with tides and in more informed circles they are known as tsunami. One such occurred in Hawaii in 1946 as a result of an earthquake in the Aleutian Islands. Waves 50 ft high struck the north-east coast of Hawaii and caused widespread damage and the loss of 173 lives. The effects were felt in Los Angeles, about 1875 miles away. The tsunami that occurred on 26 December 2004 was the most severe seismic event recorded to date. It resulted from an earthquake below the Indian Ocean and affected coastal areas in India, Thailand, Indonesia, Sri Lanka and East Africa. It is estimated to have caused the loss of over 200 000 lives and physical damage whose cost will be difficult to count. This was a case where timely warning could have saved many lives and appropriate arrangements are (in early 2005) being considered.

Liquefaction

Where the ground consists of fine grains, sand or silt saturated with water, earthquake vibration may cause it to liquefy. The foundations of buildings then lose some or all of their support. As a result they may tilt or capsize. In 1964 there was an earthquake of magnitude 7.5 with an epicentre about 35 miles from the city of Niigata, Japan. The ground acceleration in the city was about $0.1\,g$, not enough to cause serious structural damage, but part of the residential area was built on the sandy soil of a river plain and there was a high water table. This soil liquefied. Figure 6.11 shows how structures collapsed or tilted during the Luzon earthquake.

In 1976 there was a catastrophic earthquake measuring 7.8 on the Richter scale in north-east China. About a quarter of a million people died in this disaster. The epicentre was near the city of Tangshan and damage extended as far as Tianjin, 125 miles away. This part of China is low-lying and the water table is high. It was estimated that the soil liquefied over an area of several thousand square miles. There was devastating loss of life in Tangshan and the surrounding area. This was, of course, caused by structural damage, not liquefaction. In 1980 a large number of people in Tianjin were still living in brick shacks which had been put up along the roadsides as temporary housing. In rural areas the earthquake formed spouts of mud which spread over the countryside, ruining the harvest.

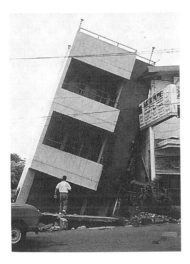

6.11 Tilted building in Dagupan, the Philippines. This was the result of liquefaction during the Luzon earthquake of 1990.

Earthquake-resistant buildings

There is no such thing as an earthquake-proof building, but a great deal can be done to minimise the risk of damage and loss of life by designing buildings that have sufficient strength to resist the forces generated by earthquakes and sufficient ductility to absorb the energy of the oscillation without cracking or collapse.

The design techniques used for earthquake-resistant buildings have developed from relatively simple formulae used in the early part of the twentieth century to the complex and sophisticated codes that are in use today. In Japan earthquake-resistant buildings had been designed and constructed by the time of the 1923 Kwanto earthquake in the Tokyo region and were reported to have performed quite well. Similar developments came rather later in California and Europe. Japan and the state of California are world leaders in the field, but their approaches to the problems, although similar to start with, have diverged in recent years.

Green[4] gives an excellent account of the way in which the Californian seismic codes have developed. The initial impetus was provided by the Long Beach earthquake in 1933. This caused extensive damage not only at Long Beach but also in the Los Angeles area. The most shocking aspect of this incident, however, was that it caused severe damage to school buildings. The earthquake occurred at 6 am, and it was evident that had it taken place during school hours many children would have been killed. In consequence the state legislature passed acts that, amongst other things, set up requirements for a building code to cover earthquake-resistant structures. These requirements were then incorporated in the building code for the city of Los Angeles.

This code, and its subsequent developments, was based on the notion that as a result of the accelerations associated with an earthquake, the building would be subject to shear forces and that such forces could be treated as static loads. The shear force is given by

$$F = CW \hspace{4cm} [6.2]$$

where F is the force, C is the seismic coefficient and W the weight of the structure. No attempt was made to obtain the seismic coefficient from measured accelerations; rather it was (and still is) regarded as an empirical figure derived from experience with earthquakes and their effect on buildings. Initially it was assigned the value of 0.08, except for schools where it was increased to 0.10.

In the case of taller buildings the use of a single coefficient at all levels is not appropriate. The deflection of a multistorey structure is greatest at the top and the acceleration increases correspondingly. Therefore the seismic coefficient must be greater for the upper storeys. In 1943 the code was modified to recognise this fact and in 1957 it was further modified because in that year Los Angeles city allowed, for the first time, the construction of buildings having more than 13 storeys. The seismic coefficient became

$$C = \frac{4.6\,S}{N + 0.9\,(S-8)100}$$

[6.3]

where N is the number of storeys above the one under consideration and S is the total number of storeys, except that $S = 13$ for buildings of less than 13 storeys.

At about the time that this formula was incorporated in the city building code, work started on a more comprehensive design technique. The deflection of tall buildings is affected by their natural frequency of vibration. Generally speaking, the taller the building, the lower the natural frequency and the deflections and shear forces are correspondingly lower. There are approximate formulae for calculating the vibration period of a building based on its dimensions. So it is possible to make a preliminary assessment using such approximations and then to carry out a full dynamic analysis to refine the design. Current practice is to carry out such dynamic analyses for all major buildings.

An important innovation at this time was the requirement that the framework of buildings should be ductile. It was recognised that in severe earthquakes the displacements could be large, so the intention was that under such conditions members should bend and not break. At the time it was considered that this condition would be met without reservation by steel-framed construction, but questionably so for reinforced concrete. Nevertheless it was argued that by providing the right sort of reinforcement, concrete could be rendered ductile. 'Ductile' concrete frames were therefore included in the code.

The brittle failure of steel space frame members in the Northridge earthquake of 1994 and at Kobe in 1995 have called some of these assumptions about steel-framed buildings into question. A good deal of work will be required to resolve this problem.

Actual shear forces

Green[4] has considered the anomalous behaviour of the Holiday Inn building during the San Fernando earthquake. This was a reinforced concrete-framed structure and it suffered the highest measured acceleration, equal to $0.27\,g$ at ground level and $0.4\,g$ at roof level.

Nevertheless, the structural damage was slight and easily repaired. Calculations were made using the measured accelerations of the shear force at the base of the building. These turned out to be $3\frac{1}{2}$ times the value used in the design of the structure, sufficient, it might be thought, to produce a total collapse. One suggestion (which is by no means universally accepted) is that materials behave differently in high-speed dynamic loading than in a low-strain rate laboratory test. Such differences have already been noted for several cases of dynamic loading earlier in the book. It was also noted that the high acceleration was of a very brief duration, so possibly the cracks did not have time to propagate across the complete section of the members.

Japanese developments[5]

Japan is located in one of the most seismically active parts of the world. It lies in a region where the Indonesian and Pacific plates move north along the Eurasian plate. The whole region is under pressure and a complex system of faults results in frequent tremors and earthquakes. There were no less than four substantial earthquakes between 28 December 1994 and 17 January 1995, the last being the Kobe earthquake, which was discussed earlier.

Japanese engineers have for the most part used the same methods as those described above for designing earthquake-resistant structures. In the late 1960s, however, new ideas were put forward and some of these, notably base isolation, have been put into practice.

The general approach has been to find means of damping the oscillations of buildings exposed to earthquake shock and to eliminate the possibility of resonance. The simplest device is base isolation, a system first developed and put into use in New Zealand. This consists of a pad of laminated rubber, on which the foundations of the building rest. Lateral movement of the pad reduces the amount of shake to which the building is exposed and tends to damp any oscillations. Californian engineers tend to regard this device as too costly to be used other than as a last resort, but of course such costs must be set against the repair or replacement costs following an earthquake.

Other passive devices are sketched in Fig. 6.12. The first of these incorporates a flexible frame at ground level which would reduce shear stresses at the upper floors. Figure 6.12(c) has a damping device consisting of a weight attached to a spring at roof level and (d) has a brace containing an oil cylinder running across the ground floor frame. A number of other methods of damping using hydraulic systems have been proposed.

The most ambitious project, however, is the intelligent building. A large movable weight is located on the roof and the motions of this weight are

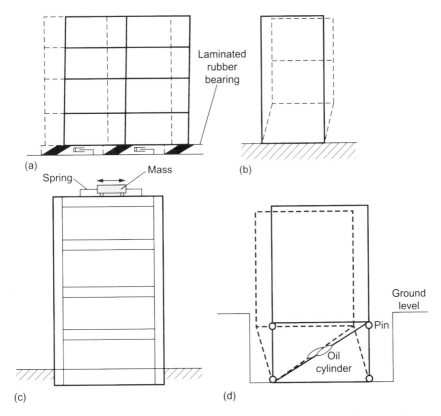

6.12 Japanese proposals for earthquake-resistant buildings: (a) base isolation; (b) flexible first storey; (c) dynamic damper; (d) viscous damper.

controlled by a computer in such a way as to counter the vibrations due to the earthquake (Fig. 6.13). There are two versions. One employs a remote sensor, which transmits a record of the seismic motions to the computer before it has reached the building. The computer recognises the form of the vibrations and is prepared to initiate the appropriate movement of the weight as soon as the earthquake arrives. The other type has a feedback loop, such that there is a response to counter any motion of the building itself. A number of intelligent earthquake-resistant buildings have been constructed in Japan.

Do the preventative measures work?

In general terms the preventative measures do work. Detailed comparisons are lacking. However, during the first half of this century, the average number of fatalities per earthquake in the developed and undeveloped

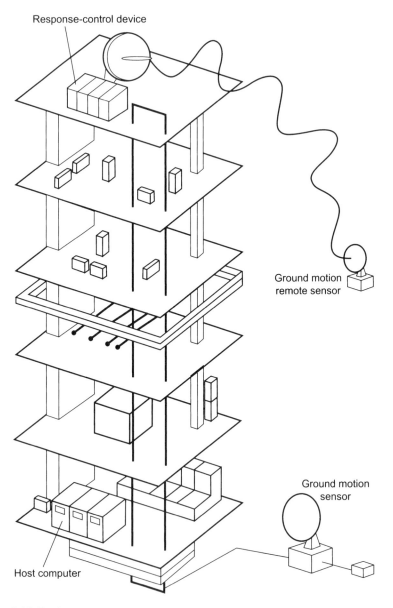

Response-control device

Ground motion
remote sensor

Ground motion
sensor

Host computer

6.13 Earthquake-resistant   building   with   computer-controlled   dynamic
response: the intelligent building.

countries of the world were about equal, the numbers in both cases being about 12 000. In the period 1950–92, however, the death rate in the developed countries fell to 1200 per earthquake (equivalent to an annual decrement of about 7%), whilst in the undeveloped world the figure remained at about 12 000.[2] There is little doubt that the improvement in developed countries was due to improved buildings.

References

1. International Federation of Red Cross and Red Crescent Societies, *World Disasters Report*, Oxford University Press, Oxford, 1998.
2. Anon, 'Major disasters around the world 1963–1992', United Nations Conference, *Natural Disaster Reduction*, Yokohama, 1994.
3. Gubbins D. *Seismology and Plate Tectonics*, Cambridge University Press, Cambridge, 1990.
4. Green N.B. *Earthquake Resistant Building Design and Construction*, Elsevier, New York, 1987.
5. Anon, *Technological Development of Earthquake Resistant Structures*, Japan Building Centre (English trans.).

Appendix 1: Mathematical models and statistical methods for accident data

The trend curve

In the normal case the accident rate falls with time and may be represented by a trend curve where the annual proportional gradient is constant. If this constant is designated b,

$$\frac{1}{r}\frac{dr}{dt} = b \qquad\qquad\qquad\qquad \text{[A.1]}$$

Separating variables and integrating

$$\ln r = bt + \text{constant} \qquad\qquad\qquad\qquad \text{[A.2]}$$

which leads to

$$r = ae^{bt} \qquad\qquad\qquad\qquad \text{[A.3]}$$

This is one form of the trend curve equation. The value of b is found by making a linear regression analysis of the $\ln r$ versus t data. b is the slope of the line giving a least-squares fit to these data.

Linear regression

It is assumed that the best fit for a point or a line is that for which the sum of squares of deviations of data therefrom is a minimum. Consider a set of x,y data $x_1 y_1, x_2 y_2 \ldots x_i y_i \ldots x_n y_n$.

It is supposed that the line will pass through a point $x_p y_p$ to which the least-squares principle will apply. Then, for the x data

$$S_n = \sum (x - x_p)^2 = \sum x^2 - 2\sum xx_p + \sum x_p^2 \qquad\qquad \text{[A.4]}$$

S_x is a minimum when $\dfrac{dS_x}{dx_p} = 0$, so

$$2\sum x - 2\sum x_p = 2\sum x - 2Nx_p = 0 \qquad\qquad \text{[A.5]}$$

where N is the total number of data. Hence

$$x_p = \frac{1}{N} \sum x = \bar{x} \qquad\qquad [A.6]$$

where $\bar{x}$ is the arithmetic mean of all x data. A similar argument is applicable to the y data. The least-squares fit line must therefore pass through the point $\bar{x}, \bar{y}$. If the slope of this line is m, its equation may be written as

$$y = mx + c \qquad\qquad [A.7]$$

The constant c may be eliminated by moving the origin to $\bar{x}, \bar{y}$ when

$$(y - \bar{y}) = m(x - \bar{x}) \qquad\qquad [A.8]$$

and the typical data point now becomes $(x_i - \bar{x})$, $(y_i - \bar{y})$. The displacement of such a point from the least-squares line in the y direction is $(y_i - \bar{y}) - m(x_i - \bar{x})$. The sum of squares of these displacements is now

$$S = \sum [(y - \bar{y}) - m(x - \bar{x})]^2$$
$$= \sum (y - \bar{y})^2 - 2 \sum m(x - \bar{x})(y - \bar{y}) + \sum m^2 (x - \bar{x})^2 \qquad [A.9]$$

putting $dS/dm = 0$ leads to

$$-2 \sum (x - \bar{x})(y - \bar{y}) + 2m \sum (x - \bar{x})^2 \qquad\qquad [A.10]$$

and

$$m = \sum (x - \bar{x})(y - \bar{y}) \Big/ \sum (x - \bar{x})^2 \qquad\qquad [A.11]$$

For the trend curve $m = b$. In practice a scientific calculation will evaluate b directly from lists of the r and t data.

The significance of the results obtained by such procedures may be assessed by means of the correlation coefficient, usually designated r. This is a figure which varies numerically from zero to 1, and may be either positive or negative. When r is zero, there is no correlation and data points are scattered at random. When $r = 1$ all data points lie on the regression line. For high values of r, say above 0.85, there is no doubt about the situation; likewise when it is close to zero. For intermediate values it is necessary to refer to tables which can be found in textbooks on statistics. These relate the number of data points and the correlation coefficient to the probability that a correlation exists.

Where the accident or mortality data show an exponential fall the correlation coefficient is almost invariably high, generally over 0.9. A scientific calculator that is capable of regression analysis will also produce a figure for r.

Non-dimensional forms of the trend curve equation

Equation [A.2] may be written in the same form as Equation [A.8] to give

$$\left(\ln r - \overline{\ln r}\right) = b(t - \bar{t}) \tag{A.12}$$

where

$$\overline{\ln r} = 1/N \left(\ln r_1 + \ln r_2 \cdots + \ln r_N\right)$$
$$= \ln(r_1 \times r_2 \times \cdots \times r_N)^{\frac{1}{N}}$$
$$= \ln \bar{\bar{r}} \tag{A.13}$$

where $\bar{\bar{r}}$ is the geometric mean of the data.
Hence

$$r/\bar{\bar{r}} = e^{b(t - \bar{t})} \tag{A.14}$$

Consider a period starting with time t_0 and casualty rate r_0 and finishing at time t_1 and rate r_1, then from either equation [A.3] or Equation [A.14]

$$r_1/r_0 = e^{b(t_1 - t_0)} \tag{A.15}$$

and

$$b = \frac{1}{(r_1 - t_0)} \ln^{\frac{r_1}{r_0}} \tag{A.16}$$

Equation [A.16] may be used to obtain a quick estimate for b provided that the time interval is greater than 10 years.

Casualty numbers

Suppose that, for a particular industry or mode of transport an exponential fall in the fatality rate has been established, then the annual numbers of deaths is qr, where q is the size of the relevant population and r is the fatality rate. Suppose further that the population grows in a linear manner, such that $q = ct + d$. Then annual deaths are

$$n = (ct + d)ae^{bt} \tag{A.17}$$

This equation generates a humped curve with a maximum at $t = -1/b - d/c$. Figure A.1 shows a plot for annual deaths due to accidents on British roads. The data plotted, and those used for circulating the trend curve, are for the years 1934–38 and 1946–2001. The peak of the theoretical curve occurs in 1960. Agreement after this date is good, but not so for pre-war and immediate post-war years.

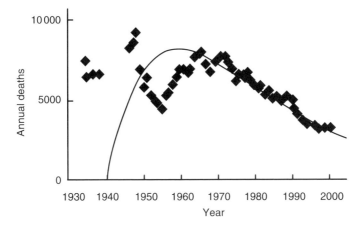

A.1 Annual number of deaths due to accidents on British roads 1934–2001, omitting data for the war period.

Hyperbolic models

An equation having the form

$$y = a/x^n \qquad \text{[A.18]}$$

may provide a useful model when the two related variables are both **finite** and greater than zero. This was the case for the relationship between fatality rate in road accidents and per capita gross domestic product, as reported in Chapter 1. The model is not applicable when the independant variable is time. This is because the proportional gradient varies hyperbolically with time. From Equation [A.18]

$$\frac{1}{y}\frac{dy}{dx} = -n/x \qquad \text{[A.19]}$$

In the case of a falling accident or mortality rate, the proportional gradient is constant or varies slowly with time. A hyperbolic model is inappropriate.

Variance

The standard definition of variance is

$$[\text{VAR}] = \sigma^2 = 1/N \sum (r - \bar{r})^2 \qquad \text{[A.20]}$$

where [VAR] is the variance, σ is the standard deviation, N the total number of items, r the measure of a typical item and $\bar{r}$ the arithmetic mean of all such measures. It is also possible to define a non-dimensional or relative form of the variance

$$[\text{VAR}]_r = \sigma_r^2 = 1/N \sum (r - \bar{r})^2 / \bar{r}^2$$
$$= 1/N \sum (r/\bar{r} - 1)^2 \qquad [\text{A.21}]$$

For the normal case of accident rate data, where the accident rate falls exponentially with time, the variation of interest is that relative to the trend curve. Also it is found empirically that the spread of data for any given year is proportional to the trend curve value for that year. Therefore it is possible to eliminate the time dimension and obtain a set of comparable data r_1/r_{t1}, $r_2/r_{t2} \ldots r_i/r_{ti} \ldots r_n/r_{tn}$, where r_i is the accident rate for year i and r_{ti} is the trend curve value for that year. The proportional deviations from the trend curve are $(r_i = r_{ti})/r_{ti} = (r_i/r_{ti} - 1)$ etc. It will be convenient to designate r_i/r_{ti} as x_i, so the deviations are $(x_i - 1)$ etc. The relative variance is now

$$[\text{VAR}]_r = \sigma_r{}^2 = 1/N \sum_{i=1}^{N} (x_i - 1)^2 \qquad [\text{A.22}]$$

The Gaussian frequency distribution

The mathematician Gauss found that the distribution of errors in astronomical observations could be represented by the expression

$$f = Ae^{-p^2} \qquad [\text{A.23}]$$

where A is a constant and p is a non-dimensional parameter which, in the case of accident rate, is

$$p = (r - \bar{r})/a \qquad [\text{A.24}]$$

a being a constant.
This quantity may range from $-\infty$ through zero, when $r = \bar{r}$ to $+\infty$. f is the frequency density gradient

$$f = 1/N \, dn/dp \qquad [\text{A.25}]$$

and is the rate of change of the proportion n/N of data numbers per unit of p.
Now, self-evidently

$$\int_{-\infty}^{\infty} 1/N \, dn/dp \, dp = 1 \qquad [\text{A.26}]$$

whilst from tables of definite integrals

$$\int_{-\infty}^{\infty} e^{-p^2} dp = \sqrt{\pi} \qquad [\text{A.27}]$$

so that the constant A in Equation [A.23] is $1/\sqrt{\pi}$. Further, the variance for data so distributed is

$$\sigma^2 = 1/N \int_{-\infty}^{\infty} (r - \bar{r})^2 \, dn/dp \, dp = 1/\sqrt{\pi} \int_{-\infty}^{\infty} a^2 p^2 e^{-p^2} \, dp \qquad [A.28]$$

Now, again using tables of definite integrals

$$\int_{-\infty}^{\infty} p^2 e^{-p^2} \, dp = \sqrt{\pi}/2 \qquad [A.29]$$

so $a^2 = 2\sigma^2$ and $p = (r - \bar{r})/\sqrt{2}\sigma$

The spread of data

The proportion of data having p values between $-p_1$ and $+p_1$, is

$$n/N = \int_{-p_1}^{p_1} (dn/dp) dp = 1/\sqrt{\pi} \int_{-p_1}^{p_1} e^{-p^2} \, dp \qquad [A.30]$$

This quantity is numerically equal to the error function, erf$p$, values of which are listed in mathematical tables. Alternatively it may be calculated from

$$\text{erf} p = 2/\sqrt{\pi} \sum_{n=0}^{\infty} (-1)^n \, p^{2n+1}/(2n+1)n! \qquad [A.31]$$

For the p values of interest here this series converges rapidly.

Putting $(r - \bar{r}) = 2\sigma$, we have $p = \sqrt{2}$, and $n/N = \text{erf} \sqrt{2}$, the value of which is 0.9545. Thus, 95% of data points lie between the $\pm 2\sigma$ limits provided that the distribution is Gaussian. This is generally so for accident and all-cause mortality rates where these decline when plotted against time. Figure A.2 is the relevant plot for the annual proportional loss of commercial jet aircraft from the world fleet for the years 1964–2002. The solid line is a plot of Equation [A.23]. The ordinates are values of $\dfrac{1}{N}\dfrac{\Delta n}{\Delta p}$ and are plotted at the middle of the Δp range.

The procedure is:

1 Calculate the set of p values from the rate data using $p = (r - \bar{r})/\sqrt{2}\sigma$ $= (x - 1)/\sqrt{2}\sigma_r$
2 Establish Δp; in this instance 0.5 was chosen.
3 List the values in ascending order.
4 Count the number of data between the relevant p values: in this instance -1.75 to -1.25, -1.25 to -0.75, . . . , 1.25 to 1.75.
5 Divide the resulting list by $(N \times \Delta p)$: in this case (39×0.5).
6 Plot the results against the Δp midpoints; in this example -1.5, -1, -0.5, 0, 0.5, 1, 1.5.

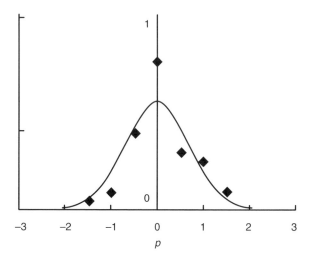

A.2 Frequency density gradient as a function of the parameter p for the annual proportional loss of commercial jet aircraft from the world fleet, 1964–2002.

Jet aircraft losses conform surprisingly well to the Gaussian pattern; in particular, the proportion of data falling between $\pm 2\sigma$ is 0.9487, compared with the theoretical value of 0.9545.

It was noted in Chapter 1 that plots of accident and economic growth rate against time show a cyclic tendency. Where this is so, the frequency distribution may show a double peak with a depression at $p = 0$. This distortion is however normally confined to the region $p = \pm 1$ and the rule that 95% of data are confined within the $\pm 2\sigma$ boundaries remains true.

The neutral case

The frequency distribution of the linear components of the velocities of gas molecules (discussed in Chapter 1) is given by

$$f = \frac{1}{\sqrt{\pi}}\mathrm{e}^{-v^2/v_0^2} \tag{A.32}$$

so that in this instance $p = v/v_0$. Also $p = (v - \bar{v})/\sqrt{2}\sigma$. The gas is assumed to be at rest, so $\bar{v} = 0$. Hence $\sigma = v_0/\sqrt{2}$ and relative standard deviation is $\sigma/v_0 = 1/\sqrt{2}$. The same result is obtained by evaluating the variance:

$$[\mathrm{VAR}] = \sigma^2 = 1/N \int_{-\infty}^{\infty} v^2 (\mathrm{d}n/\mathrm{d}p)\mathrm{d}p = \frac{v_0^2}{\sqrt{\pi}} \int_{-\infty}^{\infty} p^2 \mathrm{e}^{-p^2} \mathrm{d}p = \frac{v_0^2}{2} \tag{A.33}$$

In these expression v_0 is constant and corresponds to the thermal energy of the gas:

$$\frac{1}{2}Mv_0^2 = RT$$

and

$$v_0 = \sqrt{\frac{2RT}{M}} \qquad\qquad [A.34]$$

where M is the molecular weight, R is the gas constant and T is the temperature in degrees Kelvin.

In the present context, the neutral case is significant in that when the frequency distribution is plotted against the linear component of molecular velocity it complies exactly with the bell-shaped curve shown in Fig. A.1. If the relative standard deviation is less than $1/\sqrt{2}$, then a plot of frequency distribution against the raw data $(r - \bar{r})$ will generate a curve that is relatively more peaked, with the data points clustering more closely around the trend curve. In the text this condition has been regarded as symptomatic of a positive attitude towards the reduction in casualty rates. When the relative standard deviation is greater than $1/\sqrt{2}$, however, the frequency distribution is relatively flat and this is indicative of more risky behaviour.

A number of such exceptional cases are discussed in Chapter 2. These fall into two categories. In the first, the casualty rate rises temporarily relative to the trend curve level (during wartime for example). In these instances the frequency distribution is distorted and is non-Gaussian. The argument set out above does not apply here.

There remains one exceptional case where the frequency distribution, if not exactly smooth, is generally Gaussian: that is, fatality and loss rates in the oil industry. The record for offshore mobile craft and for financial loss in crude oil refining shows level or rising trends with a sharp fall in the early 1990s. The records in each case have therefore been divided into two parts: one before and one after the fall in the loss rate. The relative standard deviation has been calculated and the results are listed in Table A.1. Four of the six values do indeed exceed $1/\sqrt{2}$ and the other two are high.

Table A.1 Variance of casualty data for oil industry operations

Operation	Type of loss	Period	Relative standard deviation (J)
Offshore exploration	Proportional loss of mobile units	1970–89 1990–97	0.43 −0.89
	Annual fatalities per mobile unit	1970–89 1990–97	0.85 0.74
Oil refining: accidents causing fire and explosions. Weather damage is excluded	Annual financial loss as a proportion of nominal value of crude oil processed	1975–92 1993–2001	0.61 1.39

Appendix 2: Units

Units of measurement evolved rapidly during the second half of the twentieth century, culminating in the general adoption (in science and science-based technology at least) of the Systeme Internationale. This system is based on three fundamental units, the metre, the kilogram and the second. A great advantage of the system is its universality; multiplying the unit for force, the Newton, by the unit for length, the metre, gives the unit of energy, the Joule, and the same unit is used regardless of how the energy is manifest. In physics and related subjects this advantage is overwhelming but in other areas of human endeavour it is less so. For the horticulturist for example, there is no particular advantage in designating a 6 inch pot as having a diameter of 150 millimetres. Because of such considerations, possibly allied to innate conservatism, the Anglo-Saxon countries have been slow to adopt the new system.

A particular merit of SI is that it has a separate unit for force, the Newton. In earlier practice a ton for example could mean either the quantity of a substance (as in the displacement of a ship) or it could mean force (in a pressure or stress of tons per square inch). This distinction has been recognised in recent years by the use of the term ton, on the one hand, and ton-force on the other. A ton-force is the force exerted by gravity on a mass of one ton.

The table below gives conversion factors for some customary British and US units of measurements, including those recorded in this book. A more comprehensive list is to be found in the CRC *Handbook of Chemistry and Physics*, published by the CRC Press, Florida. Where appropriate here, and in the text, figures are given in scientific notations, where for example $1 \times 10^3 = 1000$, $1 \times 10^6 = 1\,000\,000$ and so forth.

Abbreviations

J = Joule = Newton-metre
k = kilo = thousand
kg = kilogram

km = kilometre
ksi = thousands of pounds per square inch
M = Mega = million
m = metre
mm = millimetre
N = Newton = kilogram-metre/second^2
W = watt = Joules/second

Conversion factors

To convert B to A multiply by	A	B	To convert A to B multiply by
9.8692×10^{-6}	atmosphere (atm)	$N\,m^{-2}$	1.01325×10^5
1×10^{-5}	bar	$N\,m^{-2}$	1×10^5
35.3147	cubic foot	m^3	0.0283168
6.1024×10^4	cubic inch	m^3	1.63871×10^{-5}
3.28084	foot (ft)	m	0.3048
23.7304	foot poundal	J	0.04214
0.73756	foot pound force	J	1.35582
2.19969×10^2	gallon (UK)	m^3	4.54609×10^{-3}
2.64172×10^2	gallon (US)	m^3	3.78541×10^{-3}
1.54324×10^4	grain	kg	6.4799×10^{-5}
1.34102×10^{-3}	horsepower	W	745.7
39.3701	inch	m	2.54×10^{-2}
2.36221	inch/min	$mm\,s^{-1}$	0.42333
0.101972	kilogram force	N	9.80665
1.01972×10^{-5}	kilogram force/cm^2	$N\,m^{-2}$	9.80665×10^4
0.101972	kilogram force/mm^2	$MN\,m^{-2}$	9.80665
3.22462	kilogram force/mm$^{3/2}$	$MN\,m^{-3/2}$	0.31011
0.14504	ksi (thousand pounds force/square inch)	$MN\,m^{-2}$	6.89476
0.91005	ksi√inch	$MN\,m^{-3/2}$	1.09884
		$N\,mm^{-3/2}$	34.7498
9.99972×10^2	litre	m^3	1.000028×10^{-3}
0.0393701	mil (thou)	μm (micron)	25.4
0.621371	mile	km	1.609344
0.03162278	MN/m$^{3/2}$	$N\,mm^{-3/2}$	31.62278
2.20459	pound (lb)	kg	0.4536
0.224809	pound force	N	4.44822
1.45038×10^{-4}	pound force/square inch	$N\,m^{-2}$	6.89476×10^3
3.61273×10^{-5}	pound/cubic inch	$kg\,m^{-3}$	2.76799×10^4
1.55×10^3	square inch	m^2	6.4516×10^{-4}
10.7639	square foot	m^2	0.092903
0.3861006	square mile	km^2	2.589998
9.84207×10^{-4}	ton (UK)	kg	1.01605×10^3
1.10231×10^{-3}	ton (short ton, US)	kg	907.185
0.100361	UK ton force	kN	9.96402
0.064749	UK ton force/square inch	$MN\,m^{-2}$	15.4443

To convert B to A multiply by	A	B	To convert A to B multiply by
0.40627	(UK ton force/square inch) $\sqrt{\text{inch}}$	$\text{MN/m}^{3/2}$	2.4614
0.16506	(UK ton force per square inch)^2 inch*	$(\text{MN/m}^2)^2\text{m}$	6.0585

* In the text this unit is written as 'inch/ton (square inch)^2'. The figure of 250 inch (tons/square inch)^2 quoted for the fracture toughness of the material of the Comet aircraft fuselage is equivalent to $39.2\,\text{MN/m}^{3/2}$.

Index